anita bean's

six week workout

BETTER BODY

Before starting this or any other exercise programme, you should check with your doctor if you have any health problems, are taking medication, are recovering from an injury or illness or if you haven't taken exercise for over a year.

While the advice and information in this book is believed to be accurate and up to date, it is advisory only and should not be used as an alternative to seeking specialist medical advice. The author and publishers cannot be held responsible for any injury sustained while following the exercises or using the information contained in this book, which are taken entirely at the reader's own risk.

Published in 2005 by A & C Black Publishers Ltd
37 Soho Square, London W1D 3QZ
www.acblack.com

Copyright © 2005 by Anita Bean

ISBN 0 7136 7198 X

A CIP record for this book is available from the British Library.

A & C Black uses paper produced with elemental chlorine-free pulp, harvested from managed sustainable forests.

Cover photography courtesy of Powerstock
Illustrations by James Wakelin
Text photography by Grant Pritchard

Printed and bound in Singapore by Tien Wah Press (Pte) Ltd

contents

Acknowledgements v

Introduction vi

1   Countdown 1

2   Exercises 11

3   Fat burning 73

4   Workout logs 81

5   Nutrition 95

6   Maintenance 101

Index 103

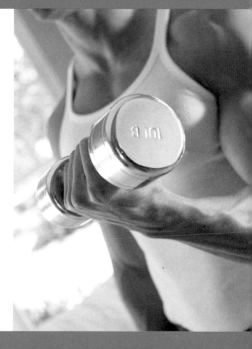

acknowledgements

Many thanks to my husband Simon, and daughters Chloe and Lucy, for all their support. A big thank you to photographer Grant Pritchard, personal trainer Steve Tunstall (www.stpersonaltraining.co.uk) for demonstrating the exercises, and my editors at A & C Black, Claire Dunn and Hannah McEwen.

Photos were shot on location at Holmes Place, Epsom.

WOODMILL HIGH SCHOOL

introduction

You want your body to look better, right? And that's a great reason for starting this six-week programme. But you'll also:

- Improve the shape of your body
- Gain strength
- Build and tone muscle
- Lose body fat
- Improve your fitness
- Perform better in other sports.

Sculpting a great-looking body takes commitment, dedication and sweat but can also be very rewarding – that's the fun part! As any athlete will tell you, there's no short cut to fitness. To get a truly better body, you need to train hard and eat smart. And that's the key: to combine resistance workouts with cardiovascular (CV) training and a nutrient-packed diet. Over the next six weeks, you'll learn how to incorporate all three aspects into your daily routine.

You'll be doing a progressive resistance programme. This means you'll be using your own body weight, barbells, dumbbells or weights machines to build strength and muscle mass. As the weeks progress, you'll add new exercises, change the order in which you do them, vary the number of sets and repetitions (reps), increase the weights – and reap the rewards!

You'll also be doing CV exercise to burn body fat – this helps define your muscles – and build endurance. It'll also keep your metabolic rate high, boost your immune system and lower your blood pressure.

benefits of resistance training

- Increased muscle mass and strength
- Stronger tendons and ligaments
- Increased metabolic rate
- Anti-ageing effects
- Reduced body fat
- Increased bone density
- Reduced blood pressure
- Reduced blood cholesterol and blood fats
- Improved posture
- Injury prevention
- Improved psychological well-being
- Improved appearance

And finally, you'll discover the best foods to fuel your muscles. Like a finely-tuned racing car, your body also requires high-grade fuel to perform at its best. By eating the right combination of healthy foods you'll have more energy for your workouts.

This motivating six-week programme is guaranteed to make you stronger, leaner and fitter. So, what are you waiting for? A toned and sexy physique is within your grasp.

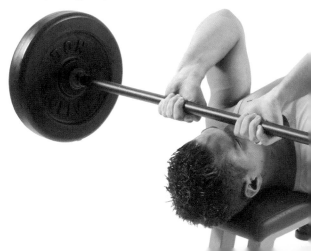

1 countdown

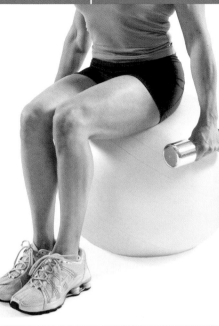

Getting fitter and leaner requires a proper plan of action. Like planning a business project or even a holiday, you need to be clear about your aims, and work out how you will achieve them. This chapter gives you the tools you need to make your plan – goal-setting and motivation techniques, effective training tips and explanations of the training methods you will be using in the coming weeks. You'll soon be ready to embark on the journey!

how to motivate yourself

Before you start this programme, you need to be clear about what you want to achieve and set yourself appropriate goals. This will help to keep you focused and ensure that you stay on course. Achieving short-term goals is rewarding and helps to motivate you towards longer-term fitness goals.

set yourself goals

First, you need to decide exactly what you want to achieve from your training programme, and why. To succeed you need to have a specific and measurable goal, such as the amount of muscle you want to gain or the chest measurement you want. Avoid vague statements such as 'to put on more muscle' or 'to get a

measuring your body fat percentage

Skinfold testing and body fat monitors are the easiest and most accessible methods for estimating body fat.

- Skinfold callipers: calibrated callipers measure the layer of fat beneath the skin at a number of specific sites on the body, usually the biceps, triceps, below the shoulder blades and above the hip bone. Ask a qualified instructor to take the measurements – the accuracy of this method depends on the skill of the tester as well as the precision of the callipers. The sum of the skinfolds is used in a simple equation to estimate your body fat percentage.

- Body fat monitor: this works on the principle of bioelectrical impedance. An electrode is placed on two specific points on the body – usually on one hand and the opposite foot or on both feet – and an electric current is passed through them. Body fat creates an impedance – or resistance – to the current, while fat-free mass permits a greater current flow. The body fat monitor measures the impedance and then uses additional information (such as your sex and height) to calculate your percentage of fat-free mass and the percentage of body fat. The accuracy depends on hydration, skin temperature and alcohol and food consumption. It is less accurate for very lean or obese individuals.

bigger chest'. If you don't know what you're aiming for, you won't know whether you've reached your goal. Measure your progress by recording details of, say, your weight, body measurements or the amount of weight lifted. See the *Body Measurement Log* below.

Next your goal should be agreed, like any contract, either with a friend or with yourself. Write it down – putting your goal on paper signals a commitment to change. Then put your written goal in a place where you can see it each day, such as on your desk or on a bulletin board. This will be a constant reminder to you and help keep you focused.

Make sure your goal is realistic – attainable yet challenging – and with a clear timescale. This programme lasts for six weeks, so set a goal that is achievable in this period. You can then go on to set longer-term goals. Write down the date when you expect to achieve those goals too.

BODY MEASUREMENT LOG

	Start	Week 1	Week 2	Week 3	Week 4	Week 5	Week 6
Chest							
Waist							
Hips							
Thigh							
Arm							
Body fat %							

achieve your goals
visualise success

Have a clear mental picture of how you will look once you have achieved your goal. Imagine what you will be wearing, how you will be feeling and what your life will be like. Visualising success is a powerful tool in achieving success. Role models can help to motivate you.

work out with a partner

Training with someone else will increase your motivation, make training more enjoyable, encourage you to train harder, cut the chances of you skipping workouts, and help you to stick to your training programme. Choose someone with similar goals to your own but not necessarily the same ability. The important thing is that you can motivate each other.

reward yourself

Decide how you will reward yourself when you have reached your six-week goal – new training gear, a meal out, a new watch or pair of sunglasses – something that will help to keep you focused and give you an incentive to keep on track.

keep track of your progress

Use the training logs in chapter 4 or buy a notebook to record your progress. Training and nutrition diaries can be great motivators during workouts. Look

training terms

Repetition (rep) One complete movement in the exercise.

Set A group of reps together (usually between 8 and 15).

One-rep max (1RM) The heaviest weight you can lift for one – and just one – repetition in good form.

Rest interval – the time taken between sets or exercises (usually 30–90 seconds).

Training tempo The time taken to complete each rep.

Overload A training load that challenges your body's current level of fitness and has the scope to bring about improvements in fitness.

back over your notes at the end of each week. If your performance matches your goals, reward yourself.

take a photo

Photographs taken before you start your new programme and then at intervals – say every three weeks – will help to give you feedback on your progress. This is more objective than simply looking in the mirror.

get professional advice

If you do not have a training partner or you need extra motivation, consider using a personal trainer on an occasional or regular basis. They will make sure that you are on track with your goals and that you don't skip any workouts, give you advice on a whole range of subjects, and help you achieve more.

finding a personal trainer

To find a personal trainer ask friends for recommendations or check with your gym for trainers who are qualified to NVQ Level 3 and have a qualification in personal training. Also check out their references and make sure they are insured. The Exercise Register (www.exerciseregister.com) lists fully qualified and insured trainers in the UK.

training tips

Training with proper form is crucial to avoid injury and maximise results. Pay close attention to the descriptions for each exercise and the following technique tips. If you are unsure how to perform an exercise, seek advice from an instructor or personal trainer.

■ Always warm up properly before starting your workout – never train a cold muscle as that increases injury risk. (See 'Warming up', page 12.)

■ Select a suitable weight that will allow you to complete the desired number of repetitions safely. Do not be tempted to lift heavier weights at the expense of good technique.

■ The general rule of thumb is to breathe out on the concentric part of the movement (when you lift the weight) and breathe in on the eccentric part of the movement (lowering the weight). Never hold your breath.

■ Use the full range of motion, taking the muscle from its fully extended position to its fully contracted position. Partial repetitions will develop strength only in that portion of the movement, and produce only slow overall gains.

■ Maintain full control of the weight throughout the movement. Swinging a weight too fast means momentum takes over to bear the load rather than the target muscles, putting your joints at risk of injury.

■ Push evenly in each movement – focus on both the concentric and eccentric phases. Resist the weight as you return it slowly to the starting position.

■ Maintain good posture and neutral alignment of your spine throughout each exercise.

■ Keep a strong core by drawing your navel towards your spine during each movement.

■ To find the correct training tempo, count to two as you lift the weight, and count to three as you lower it. Hold the fully contracted position for a count of one (but do not relax) before returning the weight to the starting position.

Pyramid Training

Pyramid training is a form of multiple-set training in which the weight is increased in each set and the repetitions are reduced. This allows you to warm up a muscle group gradually, and prepare it over the course of a few sets to cope with heavier weights by the end of the sets – hence allowing the muscles to achieve greater overload, and allowing you to develop greater size and strength.

■ Visualising your target muscle contract and relax will not only help you perform the exercise with good technique but will also help you do more repetitions

core training

Core training is the latest buzz word in gyms. It is based on the idea that by training the muscles surrounding the torso, pelvic girdle and spine – in particular, the deep abdominal muscles – you can increase stability throughout your entire body. Other exercise programmes often ignore these deep muscles but they are crucial for maintaining your posture and stabilising your spine. All movement starts from the core – or at least it should. In many cases, due to inactive lifestyles, people no longer have control over these muscles and so they develop poor posture, back problems and poor movement quality.

By training your core and learning how to 'switch on' the muscles of the torso you will improve your balance and posture by correctly aligning your body. You will also improve your performance in other sports, reduce your injury risk, and strengthen a weak lower back – as well as tone a flabby midsection. When you work to strengthen and stabilise your core, you strengthen your body's power base.

There are many exercises that challenge core stability – Pilates is one of the best-known stability programmes. Others involve exercising from an unstable

Good Posture

Find your **neutral posture**, where your joints are aligned correctly to each other:

Stand with your feet hip-width apart, knees relaxed. Let your shoulders drop down and away from your ears. Lengthen your spine and neck – imagine a string attached to the top of your head, pulling you up to the ceiling. Contract your abdominal muscles, drawing the navel in towards your spine. Adjust the tilt of your pelvis so that it is in a neutral position. You should be able to draw a line vertically from your shoulders to your hips and feet.

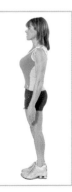

base such as an exercise ball. These place a higher demand on the deep muscles in the core as well as on your motor control system because you constantly have to stabilise yourself as the ball rolls around. They challenge your stability in many planes of movement.

There is a major focus on developing core stability in this six-week programme. Many of the exercises are performed with an exercise ball to challenge your balance and work your core muscles.

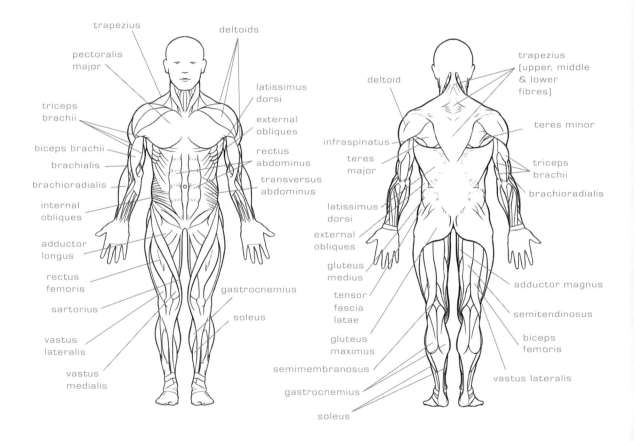

Muscles of the human body (front and back view)

Q & A - *frequently asked questions*

I've got a weak back – should I wear a lifting belt while training?

Ironically, wearing a lifting belt can exacerbate rather than prevent back problems. That's because it puts pressure on your abdominal wall, stimulating incorrect movement of your abdominal muscles (especially the *transverse abdominis*, your 'natural' lifting belt that supports the abdominal contents and protects the lower spine), leading to a weakening of the abdominal muscles. Without strong support from the lower abdominal section, the lower vertebrae are more prone to stress and injury.

A lifting belt is only advantageous when using maximal weights for certain exercises performed vertically which place considerable stress on the vertebrae, such as heavy squats and dead lifts. Even then, the abdominal wall should be drawn in towards the spine when lifting with a belt rather than being pushed out against it.

If I stop training will my hard-earned muscle turn to fat?

It is impossible for muscle to turn to fat, as it is a completely different type of body tissue. Muscle mass and strength will gradually decrease if you stop training (some physiologists believe that a muscle will never quite return to its pre-training state), and fat stores will increase if you eat more calories than you need over a period of time. However, one will not turn into the other! Once a certain muscle mass has been achieved through regular strength training, this can be maintained by training less frequently (once or twice a week).

I like to do lots of sports but I'm worried that doing too much resistance training will make me muscle-bound.

Increasing your muscle mass does not make you muscle-bound, reduce your flexibility or decrease your speed in athletic activities. On the contrary, if you train correctly – performing each exercise in strict form through a full range of motion – you can maintain and even improve flexibility.

Continuous use of heavier weights, partial repetitions and performing exercises with an incomplete range of motion ('cheating reps') usually result in reduced flexibility. Also, if you have one muscle group (such as the quadriceps) that is overdeveloped in comparison with the opposing group (the hamstrings), this can cause reduced flexibility in that opposing muscle group. This is common in cyclists and footballers due to the larger volume of work performed by the quadriceps. In any case, stretching the relevant muscles after training will help prevent them shortening and increase their flexibility.

It has been demonstrated that a strong muscle can contract more quickly and generate more power than a weak one. In fact, the physiques of world-class sprinters are very muscular, which goes to prove that increased muscle mass does not hinder your speed or your flexibility.

Will training with heavy weights harm my joints?

When properly and safely performed, strength training improves the strength of the ligaments that hold a joint together, thus making the joint more stable and less prone to injury. Impact movements such as running and jumping can unduly stress the ligaments and make the joints more susceptible to injury. The controlled, no-impact movements used in strength training, however, place far less stress on the joints than most other forms of exercise, and are therefore a good way of strengthening them.

How much weight should I use?

Select weights that allow you to complete the target number of repetitions (usually between 8 and 15). The last couple should feel hard. If 15 repetitions feel easy, you'll need to use a heavier weight. But don't pile on so much that you compromise your technique. If you cannot complete the set or you feel an intense burn in your muscles, you need to select a lighter weight. To be safe, choose a weight lighter than you think you can do and go from there.

Is it better to lift fast or slow?

Count two seconds up, three seconds down. Lifting weights too fast lets momentum, gravity and other muscles help out, preventing the target muscles from getting the full benefit. And the lowering (eccentric) phase of the lift is just as important for building strength and size as the raising (concentric) phase.

How long should I rest between workouts?

You need to rest for at least 48 hours before training the same muscle group again. Muscles need time to repair and rebuild themselves. They don't grow during your workout – they rebuild between workouts, at rest.

TIP

Concentrate on using a complete range of movement and perfecting your training technique. Don't be tempted to add more sets or push heavy weights. You need to give your body sufficient time to adjust to this type of training. Pushing yourself too hard will not produce greater benefits – recovery times will be lengthened and you may end up overtraining and risking injury.

2 exercises

Over the next six weeks you'll be doing a progressive resistance training programme to build strength and muscle, as well as a cardiovascular programme to burn fat and improve your muscle definition. For the first two weeks you will be following a circuit-based programme to work every muscle group; for the following two weeks you'll move on to a sets training system, working your upper and lower body on alternate days; and for the final two weeks you'll be training your body over three separate workouts.

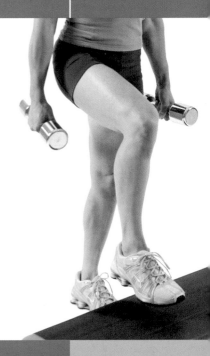

warming up

Before you start any workout, spend five to ten minutes doing light cardiovascular (CV) work – on a rower, stationary bike, elliptical trainer or treadmill – to raise your body temperature and prepare your body for more strenuous exercise. You should just break into a sweat.

Next, spend just a few minutes warming up your joints with some mobilising movements – arm circles, knee bends, shoulder circles. This helps to avoid injury during heavier training.

For each exercise in your workout (apart from during weeks 1 and 2 when you'll be doing a whole-body circuit) do one or two warm-up sets with a very light weight for 15–20 repetitions. This warms up the target muscles, ligaments and joints and prepares you mentally for the coming sets.

stretching

Stretching at the end of each workout will help improve your flexibility and posture; reduce the risk of muscle strain, joint injuries and back problems; and help reduce post-exercise muscle soreness. It will also help speed your recovery and increase your range of motion. Make sure you focus on your form and technique.

- Stretch only when you are warm. Stretching a cold muscle risks injury.
- Gradually ease into position, all the time focusing on relaxing the muscle.
- Stretch only as far as is comfortable and then hold that position. As the muscle relaxes ease further into the stretch.
- Exhale and relax as you go into the stretch and then breathe normally.
- Never go past the point of discomfort or pain. You could pull or tear the muscle/tendon.
- Stretches performed at the end of a workout should be held for 30 seconds or more.
- Release from the stretch slowly.

standing front thigh stretch

Hold on to a sturdy support. Bend one leg behind you and hold your ankle. Keeping your thighs level and knees close together, push your hips forwards until you feel a good stretch. Repeat on the other side.

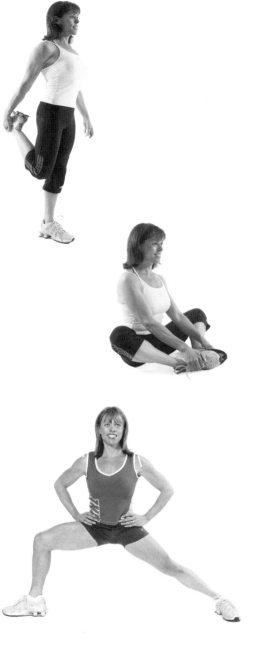

seated inner thigh stretch

Sit on the floor and place the soles of your feet together. Hold on to your ankles and press your thighs down using your elbows. Keep your back straight.

standing inner thigh stretch

Stand with your legs approximately double shoulder-width apart. With your left foot pointing forwards and your right foot turned to the side, bend your right knee until it forms a 90-degree angle directly over your foot. Hold and then repeat on the other side.

13

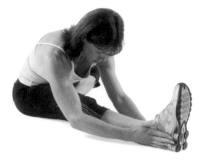

hamstring stretch

Sit on the floor with one leg extended and the other leg bent. Keeping your back straight and flat, hinge forwards from the hips. Reach down towards your foot. Flexing your foot will increase the stretch on the calf. Repeat on the other side.

hip flexor stretch

From a kneeling position, take a large step forwards so that your knee makes a 90-degree angle and is directly over your foot. Keep your body upright and press your rear hip forwards, keeping it square. Repeat on the other side.

hip and outer thigh stretch

Sit on the floor and cross one foot over your straight leg. Place your elbow on the outside of the bent knee and slowly look over your shoulder on the side of the bent leg. Keep your opposite arm behind your hips for stability. Apply pressure to the knee with your elbow. Repeat on the other side.

calf stretch

From a standing position, take an exaggerated step forwards, keeping your rear leg straight. Hold on to a wall for support if you wish. Your front knee should be at 90 degrees and positioned over your foot. Lean forwards slightly so that your rear leg and body make a continuous line. Repeat with the other leg.

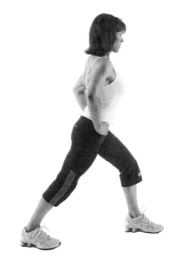

lower back stretch

Lie on your back, knees bent and arms straight out to each side. Rotate both legs to each side, keeping your head, shoulders and arms in contact with the floor.

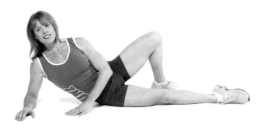

neck stretch

In a seated position, take your hand and gently pull your head towards your shoulder – i.e. your ear towards your shoulder. Apply gentle pressure with your arm over your head. Repeat on the other side.

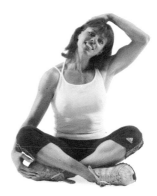

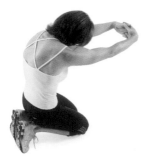

upper back stretch

Clasp your hands together and push your arms straight out in front of you at shoulder level so that you feel a good stretch between your shoulder blades.

shoulder stretch

Bring one arm across your body at shoulder height, aiming the elbow towards the opposite shoulder. Place the opposite hand on the upper arm and press gently until you feel a good stretch in your shoulder. Repeat on the other side.

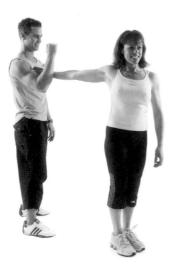

chest/biceps stretch

With your arm fully extended, hold on to an upright support at shoulder level. Gently turn your body away from your arm, pressing your shoulder forwards. Repeat on the other side.

triceps stretch

Place one hand between your shoulder blades, hand pointing downwards and elbow pointing upwards. Use your opposite hand to gently press down on your elbow until you feel a stretch in the triceps. Repeat on the other side.

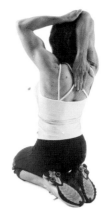

workout rules

- Aim to complete each workout for the suggested number of times per week.
- Rest for at least one day between workouts.
- If you experience discomfort, rest, then continue the workout.
- Each workout should take approximately 45–60 minutes to complete.
- Make sure you perform each movement under good control, using a full range of motion and focusing on perfect form.
- If you find any of the exercises too difficult, adapt the movement so that it feels easier, or substitute a similar exercise you are more familiar with until you develop enough strength.
- Focus on each movement – don't rush any exercise.

weeks 1 and 2

the goal

The goal of the first and second week is to develop balanced strength in the upper and lower body, and increase joint stability. The exercises are performed as a circuit – you move from one exercise to the next with only minimal rests in between. It will work all the major muscle groups in your body and build a good foundation of strength and muscular endurance. The workout contains some of the most effective movements – 'compound' exercises – that work the maximum number of muscle fibres and through a greater diversity of angles. This workout will also improve your core stability, reducing risk of injury.

■ Complete the following workout three times a week.

■ Rest for at least one day between workouts.

■ Perform 12–15 repetitions per set.

■ There are 10 exercises in this circuit. Do a single set of each exercise before moving on to the next one, with only minimum rest.

■ Do the circuit once, rest for two minutes then repeat for a total of two circuits.

■ Do each movement under good control and with good technique

exercise	reps
Warm up with 5–10 minutes' cardiovascular activity	
Leg press	12 – 15
Bench press machine	12 – 15
Machine row	12 – 15
Dumbbell curl	12 – 15
Triceps dip	12 – 15
Step-ups	12 – 15
Overhead press machine	12 – 15
Back extension	12 – 15
Exercise ball crunch	12 – 15
One-legged dumbbell calf raise	12 – 15

week 1 2

leg press

target muscles: gluteals, quadriceps, hamstrings

starting position

1. Sit into the base of the leg press machine with your back firmly against the padding.

2. Position your feet parallel and hip-width apart on the platform. Release the safety bars and extend your legs.

movement

1. Slowly bend your legs and lower the platform in a controlled fashion until your knees almost touch your chest. Hold for a second.

2. Return the platform to the starting position, pushing hard through your heels.

3. Perform 12–15 repetitions.

TIPS

- Keep your back in full contact with the base; do not allow your lower spine to curl up as you lower the platform.

- Keep your knees in line with your toes.

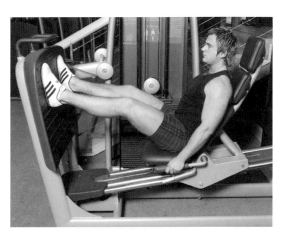

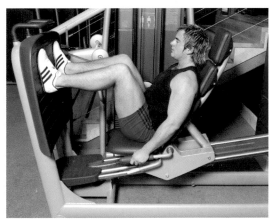

1 2

19

bench press machine

target muscles: pectoralis major, anterior deltoids, triceps

starting position

1. Sit down on the machine with your back pressed against the backrest. Adjust the seat height so that the handles are level with your chest. Depress the foot lever to allow you to grab hold of the handles.

movement

1. Press the handles away from you, fully extending your arms.
2. Hold for a second then slowly return to the starting position.

TIP

Keep your elbows at the same height throughout the movement.

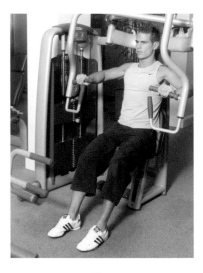

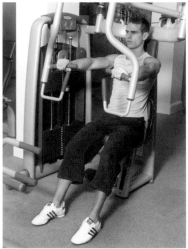

108322
613.71

machine row

target muscles: latissimus dorsi, trapezius, rhomboids, teres major and minor

starting position

1. Sit with your chest against the support pad of a seated rowing machine and take an overhand grip on the handles.

movement

1. Pull the handles towards your sides.

2. Hold for a moment then slowly return the weight to the starting position and perform the number of repetitions required.

TIPS

- Maintain the natural curve in your lower back throughout the movement.
- Don't allow the weight stack to touch down between reps.

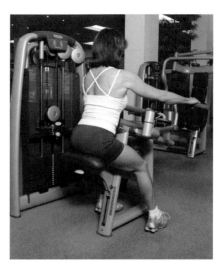

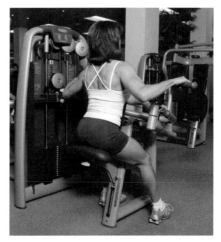

1 2

WOODMILL HIGH SCHOOL

dumbbell curl

target muscles: biceps brachii, brachialis

starting position

1. Stand with your feet hip-width apart or sit on the end of a bench or an exercise ball.
2. Hold a pair of dumbbells, palms facing in towards your body. Your arms should be fully extended.

movement

1. Curl one dumbbell up at a time in a smooth arc towards your shoulders, rotating your forearm so your palm faces your shoulder at the top of the movement.
2. Hold for a count of two; then slowly lower the dumbbell back to the starting position.
3. Repeat with the other arm and continue alternating arms.
4. Perform 12–15 repetitions.

TIPS

- Curl the dumbbells up slowly – avoid swinging them up.
- Keep your upper arms fixed by the sides of your body.

1
2

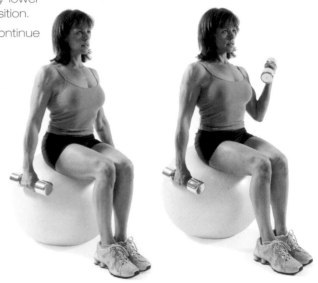

triceps dip

target muscles: triceps

starting position

1. Position two benches about the length of your legs apart.

2. Place your hands shoulder-width apart, fingers facing forwards, on the edge of one bench.

3. Place your heels on the other bench so that your legs form a straight bridge between the two benches.

movement

1. Bend your elbows and lower your body until your elbows make an angle of 90-degrees.

2. Hold for a count of two; then straighten your arms to bring you back to the starting position.

3. Perform 12–15 repetitions.

Make it harder: Place a weight disc across your lap to increase the resistance.

TIPS

• Keep your back close to the bench.

• Do not lock or snap out your elbows at the top of the movement.

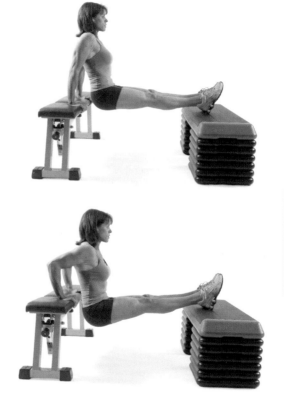

1
2

step-ups

target muscles: quadriceps, gluteals, hamstrings

starting position

1. Stand holding a pair of dumbbells facing a step.

movement

1. Step up onto the step with one leg then lift your other foot onto the step.

2. Step down with the second leg then the first. Repeat with the second leg leading.

3. Perform 12–15 repetitions.

Make it harder: Increase the height of the step.

1
2

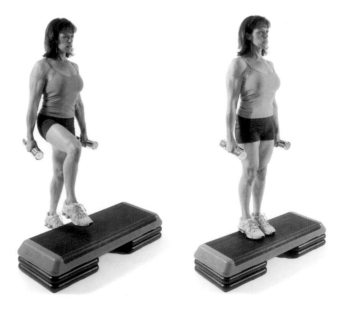

overhead press machine

target muscles: anterior and medial deltoids, upper pectoralis major

starting position

1. Sit in the machine with your feet on the floor and your back against the backrest. Adjust the seat height so that the handles are level with your shoulders.

2. Depress the foot lever to allow you to grasp the handles more comfortably.

movement

1. Grip the handles and press the weight straight up, extending your arms but not locking your elbows.

2. Lower the weight slowly and perform 12–15 repetitions.

TIP

• Keep your back flat against the pad.

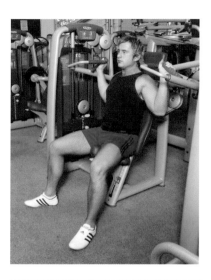

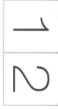

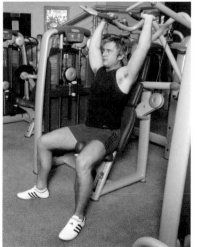

back extension

target muscles: erector spinae, gluteals

starting position

1. Lie face down on a mat or the floor.

2. Place your hands by the sides of your head, elbows out to the sides. Alternatively, your arms may be placed behind on your back.

the movement

1. Slowly raise your head, shoulders and upper chest from the floor. This will be just a short distance.

2. Pause for a count of two; then lower slowly to the floor.

3. Perform 12–15 repetitions.

TIPS

• Keep your head facing downwards to the floor in line with your spine.

• Only raise yourself as far as you feel comfortable.

1
2

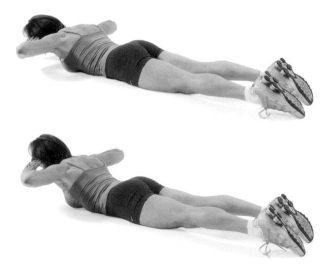

exercise-ball crunch

target muscles: rectus abdominis, transverse abdominis

starting position

1. Sit on top of an exercise ball, feet on the floor.
2. Slide forwards, rolling the ball under your bottom until your lower back is centred on top of the ball.
3. Cross your arms over your chest or, to make the exercise harder, place your hands by the sides of your head.

the movement

1. Making sure you move only your upper body and that your lower back remains in contact with the ball, slowly raise your torso.
2. Hold the position for a count of two; then lower yourself back to the starting position.
3. Perform 12–15 repetitions.

TIPS

- Keep the movement controlled when you lower yourself back down.
- Do not let your upper body arch backwards or your head flop back over the ball.

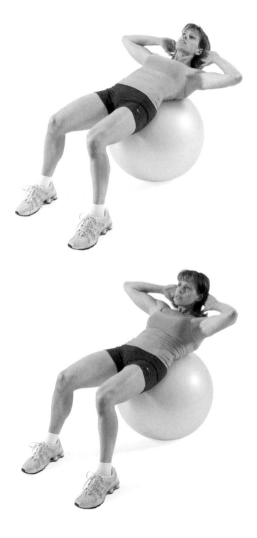

1 2

one-legged dumbbell calf raise

target muscles: gastrocnemius, soleus

starting position

1. Position the ball of your right foot on the edge of a step, allowing your heel to hang off the edge.

1. Hold a dumbbell in your right hand.

3. Hold on to a suitable support with the other hand to steady yourself.

movement

1. Rise as high as possible on the ball of your foot.

2. Hold this position for a count of two; then slowly lower your heel down as far as it will go.

3. Perform 12–15 repetitions, then carry out the exercise with your left leg.

1
2

TIPS

• Keep your exercising leg straight throughout the movement.

• Stretch your calf fully at the bottom of the movement – your heel should be lower than your toes.

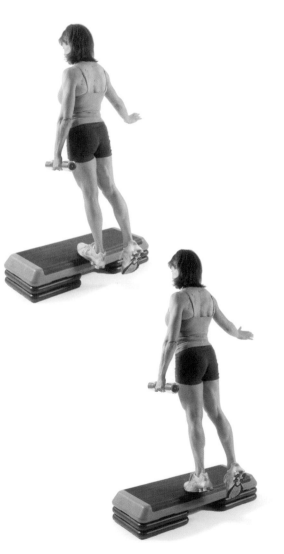

weeks 3 and 4

goal

This week and next week you'll be progressing from a circuit routine to a sets-based workout. This means you'll be doing three sets of each exercise, separated by a short rest, before moving on to the next exercise. You'll also be moving from a full-body workout to a two-way split, which means instead of training every muscle group each workout, you'll train upper body and lower body on separate days. This workout uses a pyramid training method – the weight increases and the repetitions decrease progressively with each set. In a nutshell, you'll be upping the intensity and fast-tracking towards greater strength and muscle gains.

- Alternate Workout 1 (upper body) and Workout 2 (lower body) over the next two weeks, doing a total of three workouts per week.
- Rest for 30–45 seconds between sets of the same exercise.
- Rest for approximately 60–90 seconds between different exercises.
- Use a slightly heavier weight with successive sets and reduce your repetitions from 12 to 10 to 8, maintaining strict form throughout.

workout 1: upper body

exercise	sets	reps
Warm up with 5–10 minutes' cardiovascular activity		
Barbell bench press	3	12, 10, 8
Incline dumbbell press	3	12, 10, 8
Pull-up/chin-up machine	3	12, 10, 8
Seated cable row	3	12, 10, 8
Dumbbell shoulder press	3	12, 10, 8
Upright row	3	12, 10, 8
Incline dumbbell curl	3	12, 10, 8

week 1 2 3 4

barbell bench press

target muscles: pectoralis major; anterior deltoids; triceps

starting position

1. Lie on a flat bench, ideally with an attached barbell rack.

2. If you have an excessive arch in your back, place your feet on the end of the bench or on a low step.

3. Grasp the bar, with your hands just over shoulder-width apart, palms facing forwards.

4. Remove the bar from the barbell rack and position it directly over your chest with your arms fully extended.

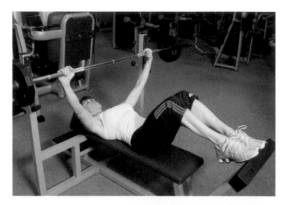

movement

1. Slowly lower the bar down to your chest. Hold for a count of two.

2. Push the bar upwards in a slightly backwards arc so that it ends up over your shoulders.

3. Perform the number of repetitions required.

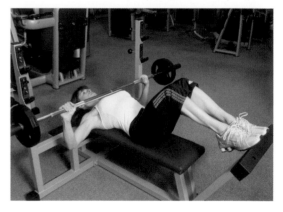

TIPS

• Do not arch your back as you push the bar upwards or you will reduce the amount of work done by the chest.

• The bar should touch your upper chest just above your nipple line.

incline dumbbell bench press

target muscles: pectoralis major, pectoralis minor; anterior deltoids; triceps

starting position

1. Sit on an incline bench, angled at about 30-degrees.

2. Pick up a dumbbell in each hand and place them on your thighs. Lie on the bench, at the same time bringing the dumbbells to shoulder level. Your palms should face forwards.

movement

1. Press the dumbbells directly over your upper chest until your arms are fully extended. Hold for a count of two.

2. Lower the weights slowly until they are by your shoulders. Perform the number of repetitions required.

TIPS

• Press the dumbbells in a straight line, not back over your head.

• Do not set the angle of the bench too high otherwise the anterior deltoids will be targeted and take much of the emphasis away from the chest.

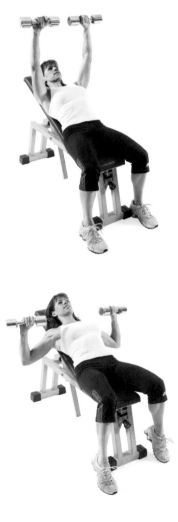

31

pull-up machine

target muscles: latissimus dorsi, trapezius, rhomboids, infraspinatus, teres major and minor; biceps brachii

starting position

1. Use a pull-up machine that has a platform to support your weight.
2. Hold the bars above your head, palms facing forwards. Your arms should be fully extended and your feet or knees (depending on the machine) on the platform beneath you.

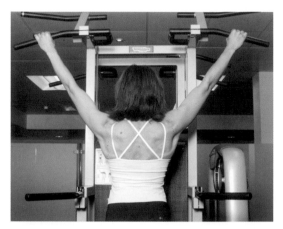

movement

1. Pull yourself up until your eyes are level with the bar.
2. Pause for a second or two; then slowly lower back to the starting position.

TIPS

• Fix your eyes slightly upwards as you pull yourself up, slightly arching your back.
• Ensure your trunk and thighs maintain a straight line.

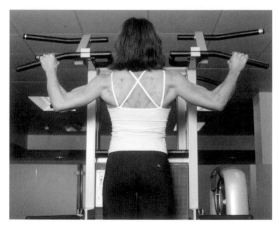

1 2 3 4

seated cable row

target muscles: latissimus dorsi, trapezius, rhomboids, teres major and minor; erector spinae

starting position

1. Sit facing the cable row machine and place your feet against the foot rests.
2. Grasp the bar and bend your knees slightly, maintaining neutral alignment in your spine.
3. Pull back a little way until your torso is nearly upright and your arms are fully extended.

movement

1. Pull the bar towards you until it touches your lower rib/upper abdomen region. Aim your elbows directly backwards as far as possible.
2. Hold for a count of two; then slowly return to the starting position, maintaining a near-upright position.

TIPS

- Keep your torso nearly upright during the entire movement – it should not move forwards or backwards more than 10-degrees.
- Do not round your back or shoulders on the return phase of the movement.

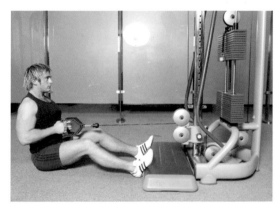

1 2 3 4

dumbbell shoulder press

target muscles: anterior and medial deltoids

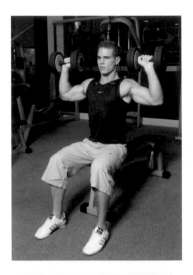

starting position

1. Sit on the edge of a bench.
2. Hold a pair of dumbbells, hands facing forwards, level with your shoulders.

movement

1. Press the dumbbells upwards and inwards until they almost touch over your head.
2. Straighten your arms but do not lock out your elbows. Hold for a count of one.
3. Lower the dumbbells slowly back to the starting position and perform the number of repetitions required.

TIPS

- Hold your abdominal muscles taut to help stabilise your spine or, if you are using a very heavy weight, use an adjustable bench with an upright back support.
- If you have limited shoulder mobility, lower the dumbbells only until your upper arms are horizontal.

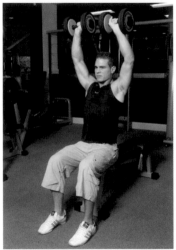

1 2 3 4

upright row

target muscles: anterior and medial deltoids; trapezius; biceps brachii, brachioradialis

starting position

1. Stand with your feet shoulder-width apart.

2. Hold a barbell with your hands about 15 cm apart, palms facing your body. The bar should rest against the front of your thighs.

movement

1. Pull the bar directly upwards towards your chin, bending your elbows out to the sides until the bar is level with your neck.

2. Hold for a count of two; then slowly lower the bar back to the starting position.

TIPS

- Keep the bar close to your body throughout the movement.
- At the top of the movement your elbows should be level with, or slightly higher than, your hands.

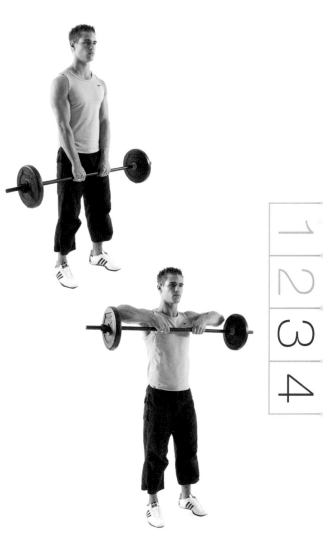

1 2 3 4

incline dumbbell curl

target muscles: biceps brachii, brachialis, brachioradialis

starting position

1. Sit on an incline bench angled at about 60-degrees.

2. Hold a pair of dumbbells by your sides, palms facing inwards.

TIPS

• Keep your head back against the bench throughout the movement to avoid neck strain.

• Keep your upper arm vertical throughout the movement.

movement

1. Slowly curl one dumbbell towards your shoulder, rotating your forearm so your palm faces your shoulder at the top of the movement.

2. Hold for a count of two; then slowly lower the dumbbell back to the starting position.

3. Repeat with the other arm and continue alternating arms.

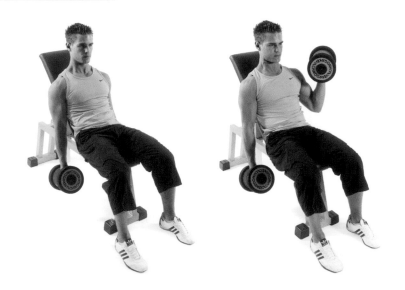

lying triceps extension

target muscles: triceps

starting position

1. Lie on your back on a flat bench.

2. If you have an excessive arch in your back, place your feet on the end of the bench or on a low step.

3. Hold the bar with your hands slightly less than shoulder-width apart, palms facing forwards. The bar should be positioned directly over your head with your arms fully extended.

movement

1. Keeping your upper arms absolutely stationary, bend your elbows as you lower the bar until it just touches your forehead.

2. Hold for a count of two; then straighten your arms back to the starting position.

TIPS

• Make sure you straighten your arms fully at the end of the movement.

• Keep your elbows perfectly still – do not allow them to move out to the sides, or backwards with the bar.

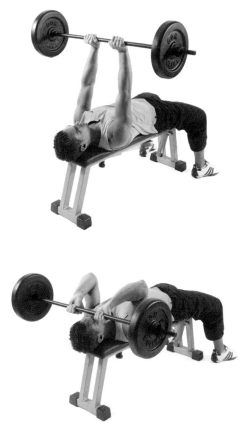

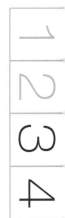

workout 2: lower body

exercise	sets	reps
Warm up with 5–10 minutes' cardiovascular activity		
Split squat	3	12, 10, 8
Leg curls on the ball	3	12,10, 8
Reverse lunge	3	12,10, 8
Standing calf raise	3	12,10, 8
Twisting exercise ball crunch	3	10–15
Side bridge	3	5–10
Dorsal raise	3	10–15

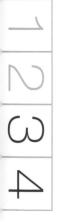

split squat

target muscles: gluteals, hamstrings, quadriceps

starting position

1. Position the bar of a Smith machine across the upper part of your back so it is resting on your trapezius muscles (not your neck). Alternatively, hold a pair of dumbbells at your sides with your palms facing your body.

2. Take a step forwards with your right leg and a step back with your left. Your left heel will lift off the floor. The bar should be midway between your two feet.

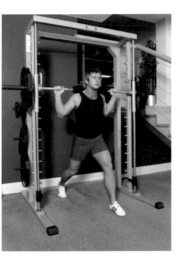

movement

1. Drop your body downwards, bending your right knee to 90-degrees, bringing your rear knee to a point just above the floor.

2. Push through the front heel to press back up to a standing split squat.

3. Complete the desired repetitions for one side, and then switch legs to complete the set.

TIPS

- When descending, think about dropping your hips straight down so you avoid bending forwards.

- Keep your head level, chest out and back straight.

- Keep your front knee positioned directly over your ankle – do not allow it to extend further forwards.

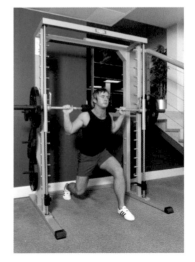

leg curls on the ball

target muscles: gluteals; hamstrings

starting position

1. Lie on your back with your calves resting on an exercise ball and your hands by the sides of your thighs.

movement

1. Using your buttock muscles, lift your hips off the floor, rolling your vertebrae off the floor one by one.

2. You should make a diagonal line from your feet to your shoulders.

3. Push down into the ball through your feet and pull the ball in towards your bottom as far as you can. Keep your bottom lifted.

4. Slowly straighten your legs as you push the ball away from you. Perform the number of repetitions required then lower your hips slowly back to the start position.

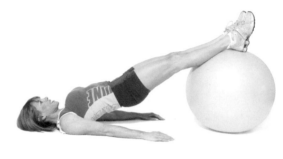

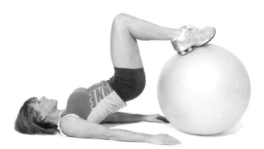

TIPS

- Keep the ball steady and moving in a straight line.
- Keep your hips lifted – they should not move up or down during the ball roll.
- Keep your neck and shoulders relaxed.

1 2 3 4

reverse lunge

Target muscles: hamstrings, quadriceps; gluteals

starting position

1. Hold a pair of dumbbells by your sides.

2. Stand with your feet shoulder-width apart, toes pointing forwards.

movement

1. Take a large step backwards with your right leg, as you bend your left leg and lower your hips. Keep your trunk upright.

2. Lower yourself into a one-legged squat position on your left leg until your left thigh is parallel to the floor. Your left knee should be at an angle of 90-degrees. Hold for a second, then push hard through your left leg to return to the starting position. Don't push through your right (back) leg.

3. Perform the number of repetitions required then repeat with the left leg leading.

TIPS

• Keep your body erect throughout the movement – do not lean forwards.

• Make sure you step back far enough so that when you lower your body, the knee of your front leg doesn't pass your toes. In the bottom position your shin should be vertical.

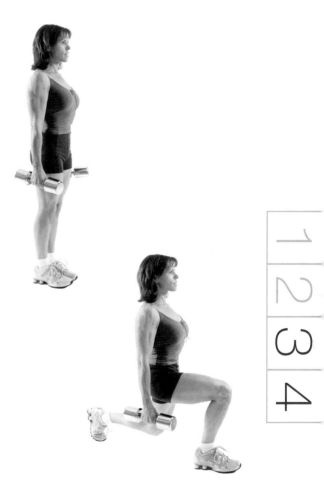

standing calf raise

target muscles: lower leg (calves) – gastrocnemius, soleus

starting position

1. Position yourself in a calf raise or Smith machine with the balls of your feet on the platform and your heels hanging off the edge.

movement

1. Rise on your toes as high as possible.
2. Hold the position for a count of two; then slowly lower your heels down as far as they will go.

TIPS

- Keep your legs straight (but not locked) throughout the movement.
- Stretch your calves fully at the bottom of the movement – your heels should be lower than your toes.

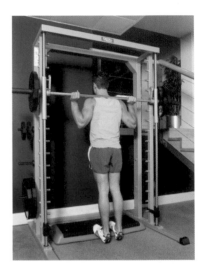

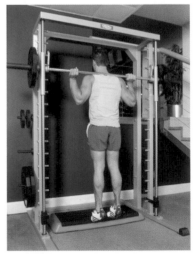

twisting exercise ball crunch

target muscles: internal and external obliques, rectus abdominis

starting position

1. Sit on top of an exercise ball, feet on the floor.
2. Slide forwards, rolling the ball under your bottom until your lower back is centred on top of the ball.
3. Place your hands by the sides of your head.

movement

1. Slowly raise your upper body, rotating one elbow towards the opposite knee.
2. Pause briefly then return to the start position, rotating your body back to its original position.
3. Repeat to the opposite side.

TIPS

• Lead with your shoulder rather than your elbow.
• Don't pull on your head – use your abs and obliques to raise and rotate your torso.

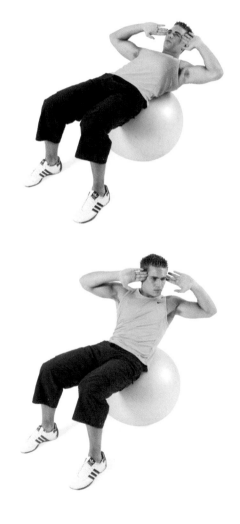

1 2 3 4

43

side bridge

target muscles: obliques, transverse abdominis

starting position

1. Lie on your right side, propping your body up on your elbow. Your elbow should be under your shoulder. Your legs should be straight.

movement

1. Lift your hips so that only your right forearm and right ankle are in contact with the floor. Your body should be in a straight line. Keep your spine long and in neutral alignment.

2. Hold for 5–10 seconds then slowly lower back to the start position.

3. Perform the number of repetitions required then switch sides.

TIPS

- Lift your hips as high as possible without rolling forwards or back.
- Keep your hips stacked on top of each other.
- Keep your neck neutral and in line with your spine.

Make it harder: Support your upper body on your hand instead of your forearm. You can raise your left (top) arm to the ceiling.

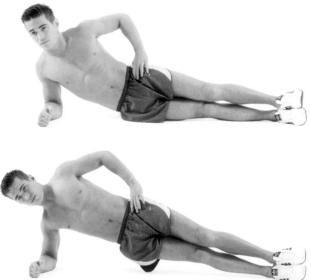

dorsal raise

target muscles: erector spinae

starting position

1. Lie face down on a mat with your arms stretched out in front of you and legs straight.

movement

1. Slowly raise your right arm and your left leg, keeping them both straight. This will be just a short distance.

2. Hold for a count of two; then lower slowly to the floor.

3. Repeat, raising the opposite arm and leg.

TIPS

• Keep your head facing downwards to the floor in line with your spine.

• Only raise as far as you feel comfortable.

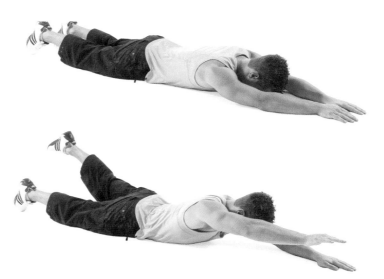

1 2 3 4

weeks 5 and 6

goal

For the next two weeks, you'll be following a three-way split, dividing your body into three areas and training each on separate days. This allows you to train each muscle group harder. You'll be doing more sets for each muscle group, which increases the total workload and stimulates greater strength and muscle gains. As for Weeks 3 and 4, this workout uses a pyramid training method. Choose a weight that will make the last one or two repetitions challenging. If you can complete 12 repetitions easily, you need to use a heavier weight. But only increase the weight when you are ready, adding 2.5–5 kg so you're able to lift only within the 8–12 repetitions range again.

- Complete each workout once a week.
- Rest for 60–90 seconds between sets and 1–2 minutes between exercises.
- Most sets should fall within 8–12 repetitions.
- Maintain strict form for each repetition, using the complete range of motion.

workout 1 (chest, upper back, abs)

body part	exercise	sets	reps
Warm up with 5–10 minutes' cardiovascular activity			
Chest	Incline barbell bench press	3	12, 10, 8
	Dumbbell flye	3	12, 10, 8
	Cable crossover	2	12, 10
Upper back	Bent over row	3	12, 10, 8
	Lat pull-down	3	12, 10,
	Straight arm pull-down	2	12, 10
Abdominals	Reverse crunch*	3	12 – 15
	Crunch*	3	12 – 15
* Perform as a superset – do the first exercise followed immediately by the second exercise. Rest for one to two minutes before repeating the superset.			

incline barbell bench press

target muscles: pectoralis major, pectoralis minor

starting position

1. Lie on an incline bench angled at 30–60-degrees. Ideally the bench should have an attached barbell rack.

2. Hold the bar with your hands shoulder-width apart, palms facing forwards.

3. Remove the bar from the barbell rack so it is positioned directly over your collarbone with your arms fully extended.

movement

1. Lower the bar down to your chest. The bar should just touch the upper part of your chest beneath your collarbone.

2. Hold for a count of two. Push the bar back to the starting position.

TIPS

• Do not arch your back as you push the bar upwards. This risks lower-back strain.

• The higher you place the bar on your chest, the greater the work placed on the anterior deltoids rather than the upper chest.

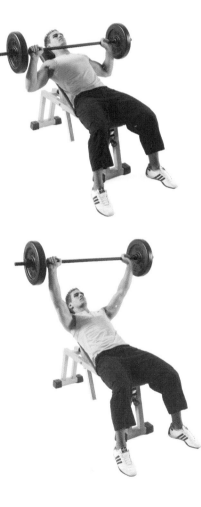

1 2 3 4 5 6

47

dumbbell flye

target muscles: pectoralis major

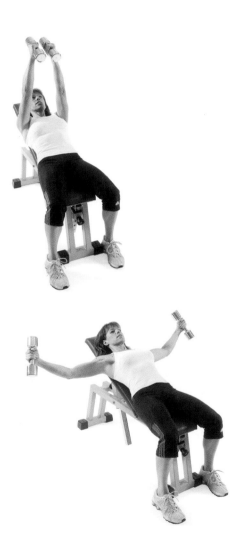

starting position

1. Lie on your back on a flat bench with your feet flat on the floor.

2. If you have an excessive arch in your back, place your feet on a step so that your knees are bent at 90-degrees.

3. Hold a dumbbell in each hand and hold them above your chest with your arms extended and palms facing each other. Bend your arms very slightly.

movement

1. Slowly lower the dumbbells out to your sides in a semicircular arc. Keep your elbows in the slightly bent position throughout the movement.

2. When your upper arms reach shoulder level and you feel a stretch in your shoulders, return the dumbbells to the starting position, following the same arc.

TIPS

• Don't allow your elbows to bend to 90-degrees, otherwise this turns the movement into a dumbbell press.

• Don't allow your upper arms to go much below shoulder level as this could place excessive stress on the shoulder joints and risk muscle or tendon tears.

123456

cable crossover

target muscles: pectoralis major

starting position

1. Attach the handles to two overhead pulley machines.

2. Hold the handles, palms facing down, and stand midway between the machines with your feet hip-width apart, or with one foot in front of the other for balance.

3. Your arms should be fully extended so you feel a slight stretch in your pectorals.

4. Bend forwards slightly from the hips and maintain this position throughout the exercise.

TIPS

• Keep your back erect and elbows slightly bent (at 10–15-degrees) throughout the movement.

• Focus on using your chest muscles to perform the movement – do not curl your shoulders forwards as you bring the handles together.

• You can vary the angle at which you pull the handles down to place emphasis on slightly different areas of the chest.

movement

1. Draw the handles towards each other in an arcing motion, aiming for a point approximately 30 cm in front of your hips.

2. When the handles meet, squeeze your pectorals hard and hold for a count of two. Slowly return the handles to the starting position.

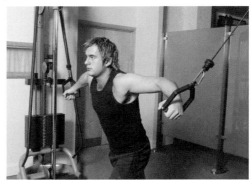

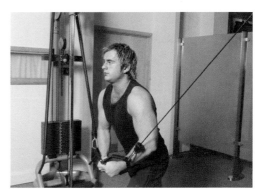

bent-over barbell row

target muscles: latissimus dorsi, trapezius, rhomboids, teres major and minor

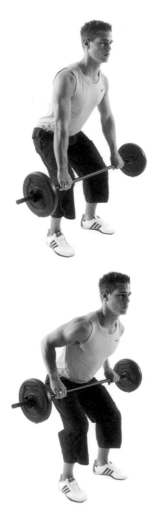

starting position

1. Place the bar on the floor in front of you. Stand with your feet parallel and shoulder-width apart.

2. Bending forwards from the hips, keeping your back flat and bending your knees slightly, grasp the bar with an overhand grip slightly wider than shoulder-width apart.

3. Lift the bar just a short way off the floor. Position your body so that your torso is near-parallel to the ground, arms fully extended.

movement

1. Slowly pull the bar towards your lower chest until it just touches the lower part of your ribcage.

2. Hold this position for a count of one; then slowly lower the bar to the starting position.

TIPS

- As you pull the bar up, squeeze your shoulder blades together and keep your elbows directly above your hands.

- Keep your back flat throughout the movement – do not round your back or you risk injury.

1 2 3 4 5 6

lat pull-down

Target muscles: latissimus dorsi, rhomboids; biceps

starting position

1. Hold the bar with your hands just over shoulder-width apart and palms facing forwards.

2. Sit on the seat, adjusting it so your knees fit snugly under the roller pads. Your arms should be fully extended.

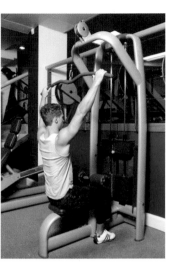

movement

1. Pull the bar down towards your chest until it touches the upper part of your chest, arching your back slightly.

2. Hold for a count of two; then slowly return to the starting position.

TIPS

• Keep your trunk as still as possible – avoid swinging backwards.

• Focus on keeping your elbows directly under the bar and squeezing the shoulder blades together.

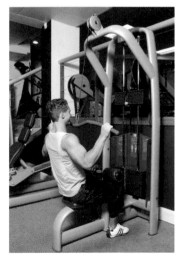

1 2 3 4 5 6

straight arm pull-downs

Target muscles: Upper back – latissimus dorsi, trapezius, rhomboids, teres major and minor

starting position

1. Stand in front of a lat pull-down machine.
2. Hold the bar with your arms extended, palms facing downwards. Pull the bar down to shoulder level.

movement

1. Keeping your arms extended, pull the bar down until it just touches your upper thighs.
2. Hold for a count of two; then slowly return the bar to the starting position.

TIPS

- Keep your wrists straight throughout the movement.
- Allow a very slight bend in the elbows – they should not be locked.
- Keep your body still and upright throughout the movement – you will need to use your abdominal muscles to stabilise your torso.

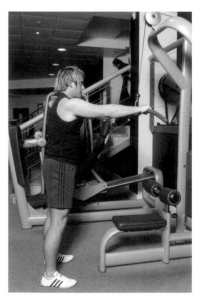 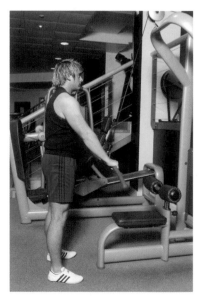

1 2 3 4 5 6

reverse crunch

target muscles: rectus abdominis

starting position

1. Lie flat on your back on the floor or on a bench with your knees bent over your hips and your ankles touching.

2. Place your arms alongside your body, palms flat on the floor, or hold on to the sides of the bench.

3. Press your lower back to the floor or bench.

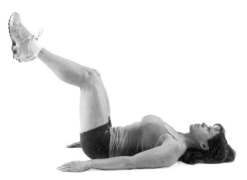

movement

1. Slowly curl your hips off the floor, aiming your knees towards your chest. Your hips should raise no more than 10 cm.

2. Hold for a count of two. Slowly lower your hips to the starting position, maintaining constant tension in your abdominals.

TIPS

- This should be a controlled, deliberate movement. Do not jerk, swing or bounce your hips off the floor; curl one vertebra up at a time.

- Do not allow your abdominals to relax at the top of the movement or while you are uncurling.

- Exhale as you contract your abdominals.

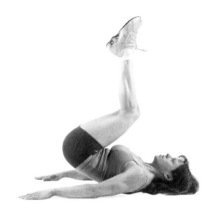

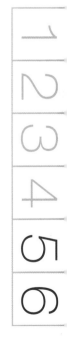

crunch

target muscles: rectus abdominis (mainly upper part)

starting position

1. Lie flat on your back, either on the floor or on an abdominal bench, with your knees bent over your hips and your ankles touching. If you are on the floor, rest your feet on a bench with your knees bent at 90-degrees.

2. Place your hands lightly by the sides of your head or across your chest.

3. Press your lower back to the floor or bench.

TIPS

- Focus on moving your ribs towards your hips.
- Do not pull your head with your hands – keep your elbows out and relaxed.
- Exhale as you contract your abdominals.

movement

1. Use your abdominal strength to raise your head and shoulders from the floor or bench. You should only come up about 10 cm and your lower back should remain on the floor.

2. Hold in this contracted position for a count of two.

3. Let your body uncurl slowly back to the starting position.

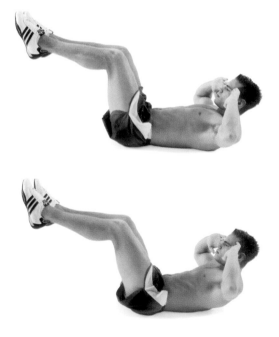

1 2 3 4 5 6

workout 2
(shoulders, arms, abdominals)

body part	exercise	sets	reps
Warm up with 5–10 minutes' cardiovascular activity and some mobility movements			
Shoulders	Dumbbell shoulder press	3	12, 10, 8
	Cable lateral raise	3	12, 10, 8
	Bent-over lateral raise	2	12, 10
Biceps	EZ bar curl	2	12, 10
	Concentration curl	2	12, 10
Triceps	Reverse-grip triceps press-down	2	12, 10
	Seated overhead triceps extension	2	12, 10
Abdominals	Twisting crunch*	3	12 – 15
	Hanging leg raise*	3	12 – 15

* Perform as a superset – do the first exercise followed immediately by the second exercise.
Rest for one to two minutes before repeating the superset.

1 2 3 4 5 6

dumbbell shoulder press

target muscles: anterior and medial deltoids

starting position

1. Sit on the edge of a bench or an exercise ball.
2. Hold a pair of dumbbells, hands facing forwards, level with your shoulders.

movement

1. Press the dumbbells upwards and inwards until they almost touch over your head.
2. Straighten your arms but do not lock out your elbows.
3. Hold for a count of one. Lower the dumbbells slowly back to the starting position and perform the number of repetitions required.

TIPS

- Hold your abdominal muscles taut to help stabilise your spine or, if you are using a very heavy weight, use an adjustable bench with an upright back support.

- If you have limited shoulder mobility, lower the dumbbells only until your upper arms are horizontal.

1 2 3 4 5 6

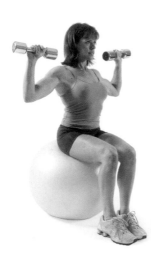

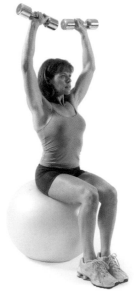

cable lateral raise

target muscles: medial deltoids (middle part)

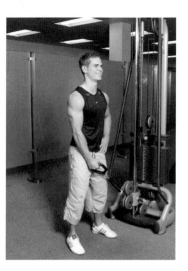

starting position

1. Attach a handle to a low pulley machine. Grasp the handle with one hand.

2. Stand with your feet hip-width apart at right angles to the machine.

movement

1. Keeping your elbows very slightly bent (at 10-degrees), raise your arm out to the side until your elbows and hands are level with your shoulder, parallel to the floor. Your palm should face the floor.

2. Hold for a second then return to the starting position and perform the number of repetitions required.

TIPS

• Your little finger should be higher than your thumb at the top of the movement, as if you were pouring water from a jug.

• Lead with your elbows rather than your hands.

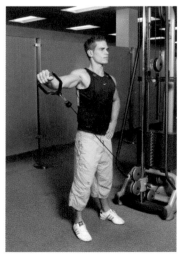

1 2 3 4 5 6

57

bent-over lateral raise

target muscles: posterior deltoids

starting position

1. Sit on the end of a bench with only half of your thighs supported.

2. Place your feet and knees together, bend forwards from the waist and hold a pair of dumbbells underneath your thighs with your palms facing each other.

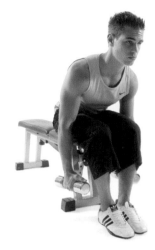

movement

1. Raise the dumbbells out to the sides until your elbows and hands are level with your shoulders, simultaneously turning your hands so they face the floor.

2. Hold momentarily, then slowly return to the starting position and perform the number of repetitions required.

> **TIPS**
> • Keep your torso still – do not lift your body as you raise the dumbbells.
> • Lead with your elbows rather than your hands.

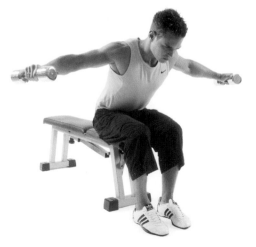

1 2 3 4 5 6

EZ bar curl

target muscles: biceps brachii, brachialis

starting position

1. Hold an EZ bar with your hands shoulder-width apart, palms facing forwards and your feet hip-width apart.

2. The bar should rest against your thighs, and your arms should be fully extended.

movement

1. Bend your elbows as you curl the bar up in a smooth arc towards your shoulders. Keep your upper arms fixed by the sides of your body.

2. Hold for a count of two; then slowly lower the bar back to the starting position and perform the number of repetitions required.

TIPS

• Do not move your upper arms or elbows at any point of the movement.

• Make sure you fully straighten your arms as you return the bar to the starting position – shortening or rushing the downward phase will reduce the effectiveness of the exercise.

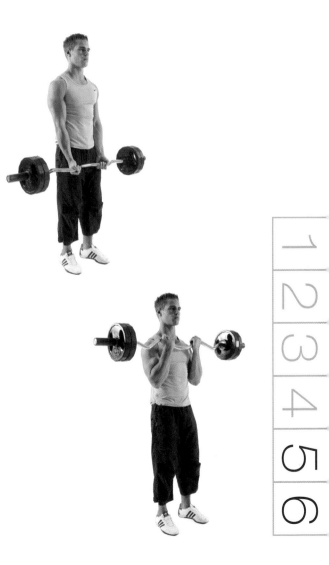

1 2 3 4 5 6

concentration curl

target muscles: biceps brachii, brachialis

starting position

1. Sit on a bench with your legs fairly wide apart.
2. Hold a dumbbell with one hand and brace that arm against the inside of the same thigh.
3. Your arm should be fully extended and your palm should be facing the opposite thigh.

movement

1. Slowly curl the dumbbell up in a smooth arc towards your shoulder.
2. Squeeze your biceps hard at the top of the movement, hold for a count of two and then slowly lower the dumbbell back to the starting position.

TIPS

• Make sure you curl the dumbbell to your shoulder and do not move your shoulder to the dumbbell. Keep your shoulder back and relaxed.

• Keep your upper arm fixed.

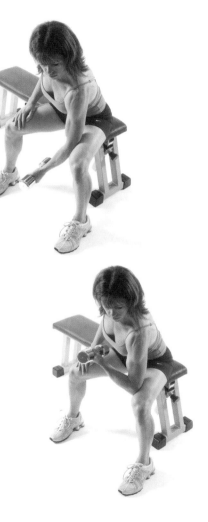

1 2 3 4 5 6

reverse-grip triceps press-down

target muscles: triceps

starting position

1. Stand sideways in front of a high-pulley cable machine. Position one leg slightly in front of the other.

2. Grasp a stirrup handle attached with a palms-up grip.

3. Bring the bar down until your elbow is bent at an angle of about 90-degrees.

movement

1. Press the handle down until your arm is fully extended. Keep your elbow in place at your side.

2. Hold for a count of two; then slowly return the handle to the starting position. Perform the number of repetitions required then switch arms.

TIPS

• Keep your upper arm and elbow locked in to the side of your body.

• Make sure you fully extend your arm and lock out your elbows at the bottom of the press-down.

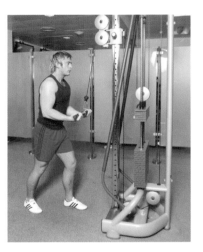

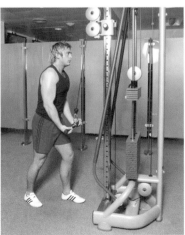

1 2 3 4 5 6

61

seated overhead triceps extension

target muscles: triceps

starting position

1. Sit on a bench, feet flat on the floor.

2. Grasp one end of a dumbbell with both hands, palms up, and raise it above your head, arms extended.

movement

1. Keeping your upper arms stationary, slowly lower the dumbbell behind your head until you feel a stretch in your triceps.

2. Hold for a moment, then press the weight back up until your arms are fully extended.

TIPS

- Keep your upper arms vertical so your elbows point directly overhead at all times.

- Keep your torso erect throughout the movement – make sure you use a weight that isn't too heavy.

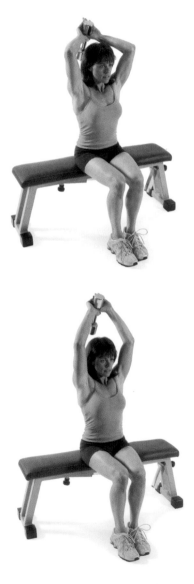

1 2 3 4 5 6

twisting crunch

target muscles: internal and external obliques, rectus abdominis

starting position

1. Lie on your back with your knees bent and feet either in the air or flat on the floor.

2. Place your hands by the side of your head,

movement

1. Lift your right shoulder diagonally, aiming it towards your left knee.

2. Hold for two counts; then slowly return to your starting position.

3. After completing the required number of repetitions, repeat the exercise on the other side.

Make it harder: As you curl up, simultaneously bring your right knee in towards your right shoulder.

TIPS

• Imagine your ribcage rotating to the side as you curl up.

• Lead with your shoulder rather than your elbow.

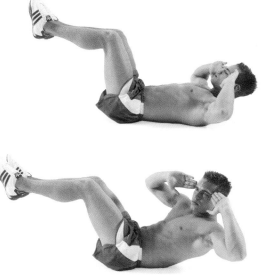

1 2 3 4 5 6

hanging leg raise

target muscles: rectus abdominis (especially lower portion), transverse abdominis, hip flexors

starting position

1. Hang from a high bar with your hands shoulder-width apart. (You may use wrist or elbow straps for support.)

2. Your arms should be fully extended and your lower back slightly arched.

movement

1. Take your legs slightly behind your body.

2. Keeping your legs almost straight, exhale and raise them upwards as high as possible. Ideally they should come just above the level of your hips. Focus on curling your hips towards your ribcage.

3. Hold for a count of two; then slowly return your legs to the starting position.

TIP

Do not swing your knees up or use the momentum of your legs – use the strength of your abdominals to move your hips and legs.

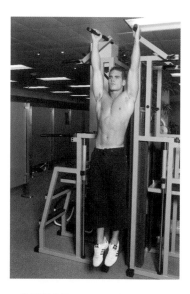

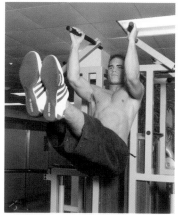

1 2 3 4 5 6

workout 3 (legs, abdominals, lower back)

body part	exercise	sets	reps
Warm up with 5–10 minutes' cardiovascular activity and some mobility movements			
Legs	Machine squat	3	12, 10, 8
	Dead lift	3	12, 10, 8
	Leg extension	2	12, 10, 8
	Straight leg dead lift	2	12, 10, 8
Calves	Seated calf raise	3	12, 10, 8
Abdominals	Exercise ball pull-in*	3	12 – 15
	Side crunch*	3	12 – 15
Lower back	Back extension with rotation	3	12 – 15

* Perform as a superset – do the first exercise followed immediately by the second exercise.
Rest for one to two minutes before repeating the superset.

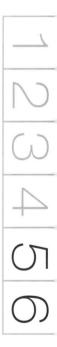

machine squat

target muscles: gluteals; quadriceps, hamstrings, adductors, abductors, hip flexors

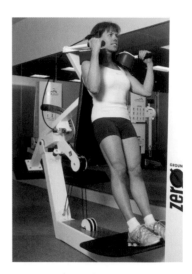

starting position

1. Position your shoulders under the pads of the machine.

2. Place your feet shoulder-width apart on the platform, your toes pointed directly in front of you, and (depending on the machine) your feet out slightly in front of your body.

movement

1. Release the safety mechanism of the machine and slowly lower the weight under control.

2. Lower your body until your thighs are parallel with the floor (approximately 90-degrees between your thigh and lower leg), while maintaining the normal arch in your spine.

3. From here, reverse directions and rise, pushing hard through your feet as you return to the starting position.

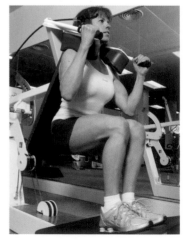

> **TIPS**
>
> • Maintain the natural curve in your back throughout the movement.
>
> • Your knees should remain directly over the feet at all times.

1 2 3 4 5 6

dead lift

target muscles: gluteals; quadriceps, hamstrings, adductors, abductors, hip flexors

starting position

1. Stand in front of the barbell with your feet parallel and shoulder-width apart.

2. Bend your legs until your hips and knees are at the same level, keeping your ribcage up and your head level. Your back should be straight, at a 45-degree angle to the floor.

3. Grasp the bar with your hands just over shoulder-width apart, one overhand, the other under.

movement

1. Using the power of your legs and hips, and keeping your arms straight, lift the bar from the floor to standing position. The bar should be against the upper part of your thighs.

2. Hold for a count of one and carefully return the bar to the floor, keeping your torso erect.

TIPS

- Maintain neutral alignment in your spine throughout the movement.
- Keep your abdominal muscles tight to support your spine.
- Drive the movement from your hip muscles – make sure you don't pull with the arms.
- Keep the bar as close as possible to your legs throughout the movement.

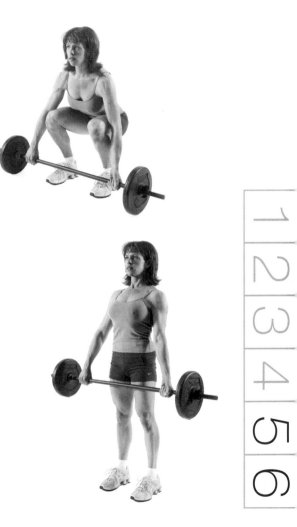

1 2 3 4 5 6

leg extension

target muscles: quadriceps

starting position

1. Sit on the leg extension machine, adjusting it so the backs of your thighs are fully supported on the seat.

2. Hook your feet under the foot pads. The pads should rest on the lowest part of your shins, just above your ankles.

3. Hold on to the sides of the seat or the handles on the sides of the machine to prevent your hips lifting as you perform the exercise.

movement

1. Straighten your legs to full extension, keeping your thighs and backside fully in contact with the bench.

2. Hold this fully contracted position for a count of two; then slowly return to the starting point.

TIPS

- Do not allow your hips to lift up from the seat.
- Make sure you fully straighten the leg until the knees are locked – do not perform partial movements.

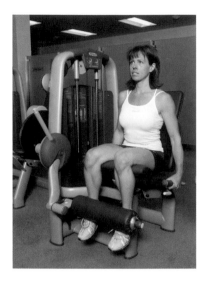

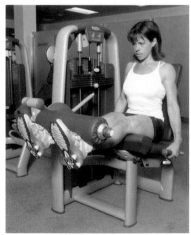

1 2 3 4 5 6

straight-leg dead lift

target muscles: back of thigh – hamstrings; bottom: gluteals; lower back

starting position

1. Grasp a barbell with your hands slightly wider than shoulder-width apart, using an overhand grip.

2. Stand up straight, looking directly ahead.

movement

1. Keep your back flat and legs nearly straight. Bend forwards from the hips until your back is parallel to the ground. You should feel a stretch in your hamstrings and gluteals. As you bend forwards, your hips and gluteals should move backwards and your body should be centred through your heels.

2. At the bottom of the movement, do not allow the weight to touch the floor and don't round your back. Hold for a count of one then return to the erect starting position.

TIPS

• Keep your back flat. Rounding your back will increase the risk of injury.

• Do not lower the bar too far. The bar should be hanging at arm's length below you, at about knee level.

• Hinge at the hips, not the waist.

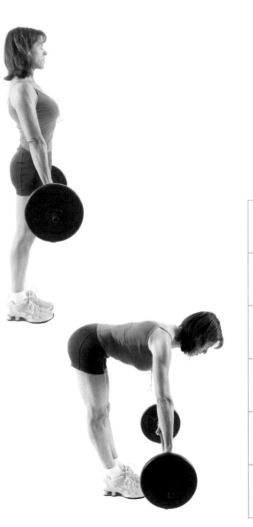

1 2 3 4 5 6

exercise ball pull-in

target muscles: rectus abdominis, transverse abdominis

starting position

1. Get in a push-up position, placing the lower part of your shins on top of an exercise ball.

2. Your head, back, hips and knees should be in a straight line.

TIPS

• Try tucking your chin in to your chest during the movement.

• Keep your back as straight as possible.

movement

1. Slowly pull your knees in towards your chest, allowing the ball to roll forwards under your ankles.

2. Hold for a moment with your abs contracted. Return to the start position by straightening your legs and rolling the ball away from your body.

1 2 3 4 5 6

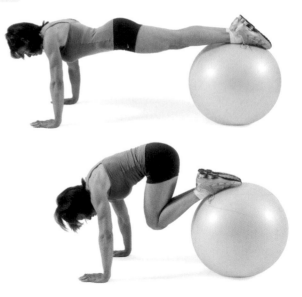

side crunch

target muscles: internal and external obliques, rectus abdominis

starting position

1. Lie on the floor or on an abdominal bench on your side with your knees slightly bent.

2. Place your top arm behind your head.

movement

1. Slowly exhale as you raise your head and shoulders a short distance off the floor or bench, aiming your ribs towards your top hip.

2. Hold for a count of two; then breathe in as you return to the starting position.

3. Perform the required number of repetitions; then carry out the exercise on your other side.

TIPS

- Don't worry if you can't reach up very far – concentrate on feeling the movement.

- Keep your head in line with your body – don't jerk it upwards.

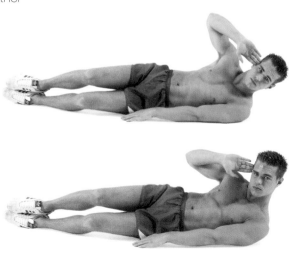

back extension with rotation

target muscles: erector spinae, gluteals

starting position

1. Lie face-down on a mat or the floor.

2. Place your hands by the sides of your head, elbows out to the sides.

movement

1. As you raise your upper body off the floor, slowly rotate, turning your shoulders to one side.

2. Return to the central position then lower, and perform the number of repetitions required.

TIPS

• Keep your head in line with your spine throughout the exercise.

• Keep your legs relaxed on the floor – do not raise them.

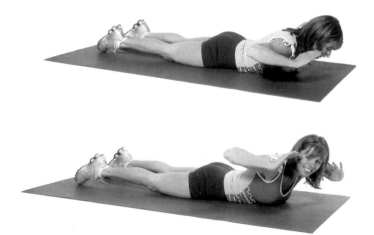

1 2 3 4 5 6

3 fat burning

Cardiovascular (CV) exercise is a vital part of any training programme. It helps burn body fat, improves cardiovascular health, helps reduce stress, blood pressure and blood cholesterol levels, and boosts your mood.

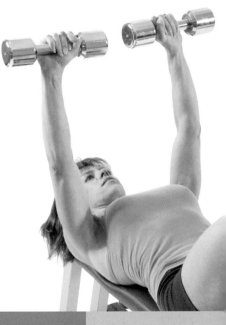

cv workout guidelines

choose your activity

Activities to choose from include:

- Running/treadmill
- Fitness/power walking
- Stepping machine/stair-climber
- Cycling/stationary bicycle
- Swimming
- Studio aerobic classes/instructor-led group exercise classes
- Climbing machine
- Elliptical training machine
- Rowing machine.

workout on an empty stomach

CV exercise performed first thing in the morning on an empty stomach burns more fat than at any other time. That's because insulin levels are at their lowest and glucagon levels are at their highest. This encourages your body to draw on its fat reserves for fuel. If you work out after eating, your body will use this food for fuel instead. Exercising first thing in the morning also helps kick-start your metabolism so you'll burn more calories during the rest of the day.

do cv exercise and weights on separate days

If you want to build muscle mass as well as burn fat, try to do your CV workout on a different day from weights. Research suggests that overall calorie expenditure is greater if CV and weight-training exercise are done on separate days. But if you have to do both in one session, complete your weight-training workout first when glycogen stores are high. Do it the other way round and you risk lower strength and muscle mass gains.

add intervals

Doing intervals – alternating short periods of high-intensity work with lower-intensity recovery periods – increases your calorie burn. It also helps you burn more calories afterwards. One US study found that doing intervals speeds up your metabolic rate up to 18 hours after your workout. Plus, intervals get you fitter and strengthen your heart and lungs more than training at a steady pace. However, it is only suitable for those with a good level of fitness to start with. Beginners should build up basic fitness with steady-pace exercise first.

Intervals can be applied to any mode of CV exercise. Intersperse faster bursts of activity, such as by increasing your speed or the resistance of the machine, with more moderate recovery periods.

measuring cv intensity

You will get the greatest benefits from your workout by exercising at the appropriate intensity level. Use this simple formula to estimate your heart rate training zone: subtract your age from 220 to get your maximal heart rate (MHR). For example, if you are 30, your MHR would be 220 – 30 = 190 beats per minute (bpm).

Consult the *Target Heart Rate Training Guide* overleaf, to find out which zone you are training in. Each zone is basically a percentage of your MHR.

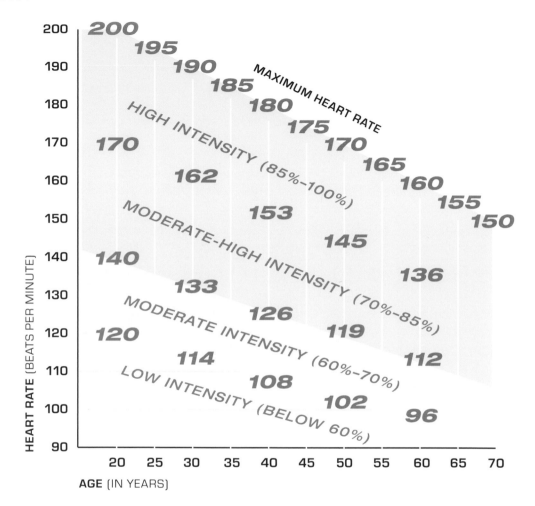

The best way to monitor your heart rate during your workout is by using a heart rate monitor, or by taking your pulse manually. Count your heart rate at your wrist or neck for 10 seconds and multiply that number by six (which gives you your heart rate in beats per minute). Check to see which target heart rate (THR) zone you are in.

Rating of Perceived Exertion (RPE)

At rest	1	Non-exercise HR
Light activity – sitting working	2	Non-exercise HR
Light activity – walking at leisurely pace	3	Non-exercise HR
Moderate activity – purposeful walking	4	Non-exercise HR
Moderate activity –brisk walking	5	Non-exercise HR
Somewhat hard activity – jogging	6	60% MHR
Hard activity – running, breathing harder	7	65–75% MHR
Very hard activity – running, conversation just possible	8	80% MHR
Very very hard activity – fast running, conversation difficult	9	85% MHR
Maximum effort – unable to speak	10	MHR

Alternatively, you can use perceived exertion (PE) instead of THR to monitor the intensity of your CV workout (see the table opposite). This is a subjective rating of how hard you feel you are exercising. It is a 10-point scale ranging from 1 (nothing at all) to 10 (maximum effort). This system correlates closely with THR, so if you're working out at RPE level 6, you are working out at about 60 per cent of your MHR.

your cv workout

Your fat-burning CV workout consists of three parts: a warm-up (5 minutes), a CV session (20–40 minutes) and a cool-down (5 minutes).

The warm-up serves to raise your body temperature, prepares your body for more strenuous exercise and reduces injury risk. The CV session should last for a minimum of 20 minutes. The cool-down allows your body temperature, muscles and circulatory system time to return to normal. If you stop too quickly, you may feel dizzy and faint.

To make improvements over time you need to progressively challenge your system. Each week, you need to work a bit harder to continue making fitness gains. You can do any of the following:

■ Increase the number of times you work out to a maximum of five per week.

■ Increase your workout time (to a maximum of 60 minutes).

■ Increase the intensity, such as your speed or resistance of the machine.

■ Add more intervals.

BEGINNERS' STEADY PACE FAT-BURNER WORKOUT

Total exercise time = 30 minutes

Exercise time (minutes)	Stage	Intensity (THR)	Intensity (PE)
5	Warm-up	50%	5
20	Steady pace	60%	6
5	Cool-down	50%	5

INTERMEDIATE INTERVAL FAT-BURNER WORKOUT

Total exercise time = 34 minutes

Exercise time (minutes)	Stage	Intensity (THR)	Intensity (PE)
5	Warm-up	50%	5
2	Interval	70%	7
2	Recovery	60%	6
2	Interval	70%	7
2	Recovery	60%	6
2	Interval	70%	7
2	Recovery	60%	6
2	Interval	70%	7
2	Recovery	60%	6
2	Interval	70%	7
2	Recovery	60%	6
2	Interval	70%	7
2	Recovery	60%	6
5	Cool down	50%	5

ADVANCED INTERVAL FAT-BURNER WORKOUT

Total exercise time = 34 minutes

Exercise time (minutes)	Stage	Intensity (THR)	Intensity (PE)
5	Warm-up	50%	5
2	Interval	70%	7
2	Recovery	60%	6
1	Interval	80%	8–9
2	Recovery	60%	6
1	Interval	80%	8–9
2	Recovery	60%	6
1	Interval	80%	8–9
2	Recovery	60%	6
1	Interval	80%	8–9
2	Recovery	60%	6
1	Interval	80%	8–9
2	Recovery	60%	6
1	Interval	80%	8–9
2	Recovery	70%	7
2	Recovery	60%	6
5	Cool down	50%	5

4 workout logs

Use the workout logs in this chapter to record your progress throughout the six-week programme. You can choose which days of the week suit you best for your workouts, as long as you take the same number of rest days between them. The days given below are guidelines only.

	day	workout	exercise	goal reps	actual reps
week 1	Monday	Week 1 workout	Leg press	12 – 15	Set 1: Set 2:
			Bench press machine	12 – 15	Set 1: Set 2:
			Machine row	12 – 15	Set 1: Set 2:
			Dumbbell curl	12 – 15	Set 1: Set 2:
			Triceps dip	12 – 15	Set 1: Set 2:
			Step-ups	12 – 15	Set 1: Set 2:
			Overhead press machine	12 – 15	Set 1: Set 2:
			Back extension	12 – 15	Set 1: Set 2:
			Exercise ball crunch	12 – 15	Set 1: Set 2:
			One-legged dumbbell calf raise	12 – 15	Set 1: Set 2:
	Tuesday	Beginners' CV workout			
	Wednesday	Week 1 workout	Leg press	12 – 15	Set 1: Set 2:
			Bench press machine	12 – 15	Set 1: Set 2:
			Machine row	12 – 15	Set 1: Set 2:
			Dumbbell curl	12 – 15	Set 1: Set 2:
			Triceps dip	12 – 15	Set 1: Set 2:
			Step-ups	12 – 15	Set 1: Set 2:
			Overhead press machine	12 – 15	Set 1: Set 2:

		Back extension	12 – 15	Set 1:
				Set 2:
		Exercise ball crunch	12 – 15	Set 1:
				Set 2:
		One-legged dumbbell calf raise	12 – 15	Set 1
				Set 2:
Thursday	Beginners' CV workout			
Friday	Week 1 workout	Leg press	12 – 15	Set 1:
				Set 2:
		Bench press machine	12 – 15	Set 1:
				Set 2:
		Machine row	12 – 15	Set 1:
				Set 2:
		Dumbbell curl	12 – 15	Set 1:
				Set 2:
		Triceps dip	12 – 15	Set 1:
				Set 2:
		Step-ups	12 – 15	Set 1:
				Set 2:
		Overhead press machine	12 – 15	Set 1:
				Set 2:
		Back extension	12 – 15	Set 1:
				Set 2:
		Exercise ball crunch	12 – 15	Set 1:
				Set 2:
		One-legged dumbbell calf raise	12 – 15	Set 1:
				Set 2:
Saturday	Beginners' CV workout			
Sunday	Rest day			

week 2	day	workout	exercise	goal reps	actual reps
	Monday	Week 2 workout	Leg press	12 – 15	Set 1: Set 2:
			Bench press machine	12 – 15	Set 1: Set 2:
			Machine row	12 – 15	Set 1: Set 2:
			Dumbbell curl	12 – 15	Set 1: Set 2:
			Triceps dip	12 – 15	Set 1: Set 2:
			Step-ups	12 – 15	Set 1: Set 2:
			Overhead press machine	12 – 15	Set 1: Set 2:
			Back extension	12 – 15	Set 1: Set 2:
			Exercise ball crunch	12 – 15	Set 1: Set 2:
			One-legged dumbbell calf raise	12 – 15	Set 1: Set 2:
	Tuesday	Beginners' CV workout			
	Wednesday	Week 2 workout	Leg press	12 – 15	Set 1: Set 2:
			Bench press machine	12 – 15	Set 1: Set 2:
			Machine row	12 – 15	Set 1: Set 2:
			Dumbbell curl	12 – 15	Set 1: Set 2:
			Triceps dip	12 – 15	Set 1: Set 2:
			Step-ups	12 – 15	Set 1: Set 2:
			Overhead press machine	12 – 15	Set 1: Set 2:

		Back extension	12 – 15	Set 1:
				Set 2:
		Exercise ball crunch	12 – 15	Set 1:
				Set 2:
		One-legged dumbbell calf raise	12 – 15	Set 1
				Set 2:
Thursday	Beginners' CV workout			
Friday	Week 2 workout	Leg press	12 – 15	Set 1:
				Set 2:
		Bench press machine	12 – 15	Set 1:
				Set 2:
		Machine row	12 – 15	Set 1:
				Set 2:
		Dumbbell curl	12 – 15	Set 1:
				Set 2:
		Triceps dip	12 – 15	Set 1:
				Set 2:
		Step-ups	12 – 15	Set 1:
				Set 2:
		Overhead press machine	12 – 15	Set 1:
				Set 2:
		Back extension	12 – 15	Set 1:
				Set 2:
		Exercise ball crunch	12 – 15	Set 1:
				Set 2:
		One-legged dumbbell calf raise	12 – 15	Set 1:
				Set 2:
Saturday	Beginners' CV workout			
Sunday	Rest day			

week 3	day	workout	exercise	goal reps	actual reps
	Monday	Week 3/4 upper-body workout	Bench press	12/10/8	/ /
			Incline dumbbell press	12/10/8	/ /
			Pull-up/chin-up machine	12/10/8	/ /
			Seated cable row	12/10/8	/ /
			Dumbbell shoulder press	12/10/8	/ /
			Upright row	12/10/8	/ /
			Incline dumbbell curl	12/10/8	/ /
			Lying triceps extension	12/10/8	/ /
	Tuesday	Intermediate CV workout			
	Wednesday	Week 3/4 lower-body workout	Split squat	12/10/8	/ /
			Leg curls on the ball	12/10/8	/ /
			Reverse lunge	12/10/8	/ /
			Standing calf raise	12/10/8	/ /
			Twisting exercise-ball crunch	10–15	Set 1: Set 2:
			Side bridge	5–10	Set 1: Set 2: Set 3:
			Dorsal raise	10–15	Set 1: Set 2: Set 3:
	Thursday	Intermediate CV workout			
	Friday	Week 3/4 upper-body workout	Bench press	12/10/8	/ /
			Incline dumbbell press	12/10/8	/ /
			Pull-up/chin-up machine	12/10/8	/ /

			Seated cable row	12/10/8	/	/
			Dumbbell shoulder press	12/10/8	/	/
			Upright row	12/10/8	/	/
			Incline dumbbell curl	12/10/8	/	/
			Lying triceps extension	12/10/8	/	/
Saturday	Intermediate CV workout					
Sunday	Rest day					

week 4	day	workout	exercise	goal reps	actual reps
	Monday	Week 3/4 lower-body workout	Split squat	12/10/8	/ /
			Leg curls on the ball	12/10/8	/ /
			Reverse lunge	12/10/8	/ /
			Standing calf raise	12/10/8	/ /
			Twisting exercise-ball crunch	10–15	Set 1: Set 2: Set 3:
			Side bridge	5–10	Set 1: Set 2: Set 3:
			Dorsal raise	10–15	Set 1: Set 2: Set 3:
	Tuesday	Intermediate CV workout			
	Wednesday	Week 3/4 upper-body workout	Bench press	12/10/8	/ /
			Incline dumbbell press	12/10/8	/ /
			Pull-up/chin-up machine	12/10/8	/ /
			Seated cable row	12/10/8	/ /
			Dumbbell shoulder press	12/10/8	/ /
			Upright row	12/10/8	/ /
			Incline dumbbell curl	12/10/8	/ /
			Lying triceps extension	12/10/8	/ /
	Thursday	Intermediate CV workout			
	Friday	Week 3/4 lower-body workout	Split squat	12/10/8	/ /
			Leg curls on the ball	12/10/8	/ /
			Reverse lunge	12/10/8	/ /
			Standing calf raise	12/10/8	/ /
			Twisting exercise-ball crunch	10–15	Set 1: Set 2: Set 3:

			Side bridge	5–10	Set 1:
					Set 2:
					Set 3:
			Dorsal raise	10–15	Set 1:
					Set 2:
					Set 3:
Saturday	Intermediate CV workout				
Sunday	Rest day				

	day	workout	exercise	goal reps	actual reps
week 5	Monday	Week 5/6 chest/back /abs workout	Incline barbell press	12/10/8	/ /
			Dumbbell flye	12/10/8	/ /
			Cable crossover	12/10/8	/ /
			Bent-over row	12/10/8	/ /
			Lat pull-down	12/10/8	/ /
			Straight arm pull-down	12/10/8	/ /
			Reverse crunch	12–15	Set 1: Set 2: Set 3:
			Crunch	12–15	Set 1: Set 2: Set 3:
	Tuesday	Advanced CV workout			
	Wednesday	Week 5/6 shoulders/arms /abs workout	Dumbbell shoulder press	12/10/8	/ /
			Cable lateral raise	12/10/8	/ /
			Bent-over lateral raise	12/10/8	/ /
			EZ bar curl	12/10/8	/ /
			Concentration curl	12/10/8	/ /
			Reverse-grip triceps press-down	12/10/8	/ /
			Seated overhead triceps extension	12/10/8	/ /
			Twisting crunch	12–15	Set 1: Set 2: Set 3:
			Hanging leg raise	12–15	Set 1: Set 2: Set 3:
	Thursday	Advanced CV workout			
	Friday	Week 5/6 legs /abs workout:	Machine squat	12/10/8	/ /

		Dead lift	12/10/8	/ /	
		Leg extension	12/10/8	/ /	
		Straight-leg dead lift	12/10/8	/ /	
		Seated calf raise	12/10/8	/ /	
		Exercise-ball pull-in	12–15	Set 1:	
				Set 2:	
				Set 3:	
		Side crunch	12–15	Set 1:	
				Set 2:	
				Set 3:	
		Back extension with rotation	12–15	Set 1:	
				Set 2:	
				Set 3:	
Saturday	Advanced CV workout				
Sunday	Rest day				

week 6	day	workout	exercise	goal reps	actual reps		
	Monday	Week 5/6 chest/back /abs workout	Incline barbell press	12/10/8	/	/	
			Dumbbell flye	12/10/8	/	/	
			Cable crossover	12/10/8	/	/	
			Bent-over row	12/10/8	/	/	
			Lat pull-down	12/10/8	/	/	
			Straight arm pull-down	12/10/8	/	/	
			Reverse crunch	12–15	Set 1: Set 2: Set 3:		
			Crunch	12–15	Set 1: Set 2: Set 3:		
	Tuesday	Advanced CV workout					
	Wednesday	Week 5/6 shoulders/arms /abs workout	Dumbbell shoulder press	12/10/8	/	/	
			Cable lateral raise	12/10/8	/	/	
			Bent-over lateral raise	12/10/8	/	/	
			EZ bar curl	12/10/8	/	/	
			Concentration curl	12/10/8	/	/	
			Reverse-grip triceps press-down	12/10/8	/	/	
			Seated overhead triceps extension	12/10/8	/	/	
			Twisting crunch	12–15	Set 1: Set 2: Set 3:		
			Hanging leg raise	12–15	Set 1: Set 2: Set 3:		
	Thursday	Advanced CV workout					

Friday	Week 5/ 6 legs/abs workout	Machine squat	12/10/8	//
		Dead lift	12/10/8	//
		Leg extension	12/10/8	//
		Straight-leg dead lift	12/10/8	//
		Seated calf raise	12/10/8	//
		Exercise-ball pull-in	12–15	Set 1: Set 2: Set 3:
		Side crunch	12–15	Set 1: Set 2: Set 3:
		Back extension with rotation	12–15	Set 1: Set 2: Set 3:
Saturday	Advanced CV workout			
Sunday	Rest day			

5 nutrition

To gain muscle and lose body fat, you need to follow a smart eating plan as well as train hard. It's important to fuel your body properly and ensure that you eat the right balance of carbohydrates, protein and fat. A well-planned diet will help give you plenty of energy for training, promote speedy recovery after your workouts and ensure your muscles get stronger each day.

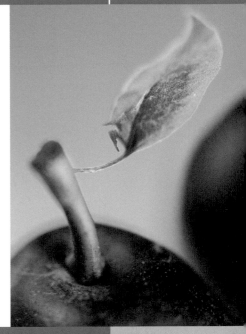

better body nutrition guidelines

eat enough

When it comes to building muscle, your calorie intake is very important. To gain weight, you need to take in more calories than you burn. Increase your usual calorie intake by 20 per cent – that works out at an extra 500 calories daily for most gym-goers.

how many calories do I need?

Record your food intake for seven days. Be as accurate as possible, recording the exact weights of all foods and drinks consumed. Use food tables, food labels or the Internet to work out your daily calorie intake. Add up all seven days and divide by seven to get a daily average. Then add 20 per cent to that number (multiply by 1.2). This will be your new calorie intake to start adding muscle.

eat often

To fuel your muscles while preventing an increase in body fat, divide your food into five to six meals a day. Smaller meals provide a steady and constant supply of protein and carbohydrates, two key nutrients for muscle repair and growth.

TIP

Smaller meals throughout the day are easier to digest and produce greater increases in fat-free muscle mass.

get your protein

Muscles need protein to help them grow and rebuild from intense workouts. Without enough protein, you may as well kiss muscle growth goodbye. Aim to consume between 1.4 and 1.8 g of protein per kilo of body weight daily. So if you weigh 70 kg, you would need between 98 and 126 g per day.

TIP

As a rule of thumb, a portion of meat, fish or poultry is 80 g, about the size of a deck of cards. For cheese, choose a size equivalent to four dice.

Chicken and turkey breast, fish, lean red meat, eggs, low-fat dairy products and protein powders provide complete protein, including the eight essential amino acids muscles need to grow. Tofu and other soya products, Quorn, beans, lentils, nuts and cereals provide incomplete protein – smaller amounts of the essential aminos – but combining two or more increases the overall protein value.

If you're trying to gain muscle mass but want to keep body fat under control, choose lower-fat protein sources like skinless poultry, very low-fat dairy products and protein powders.

fuel your body

Carbohydrates provide your muscles with fuel for lifting weights. They also stimulate the release of insulin – an anabolic hormone that drives protein and carbohydrates into the muscle cells, encouraging muscle-building.

You need to eat 5–8 g of carbohydrate per kilo of body weight daily, depending on your individual metabolism, body fat level and training volume. If you weigh 70 kg, you would need 350–560 g a day.

Choose fibre-rich carbohydrates like potatoes, bread, porridge, rice, pasta, fruit, beans and lentils. Honey, dried fruit and fruit juice are denser sources of carbohydrates and make it easier to reach your daily needs if you have a fast metabolism. If you tend to gain body fat easily or have a slower metabolism, stick with natural fibre-rich carbs, which are more filling.

TIP

A serving of grains and potatoes is about the size of your clenched fist.

get your five-a-day

The World Health Organization recommends eating five portions of fruit and vegetables a day (400g). Fruit and vegetables are rich in vitamins (especially vitamin C and beta-carotene), minerals, fibre and important plant nutrients, which help protect against heart disease and cancer, and boost your immunity.

A portion of fruit can be:

■ 1 apple, orange or banana

■ 2 apricots, kiwi fruits or satsumas

■ A cupful of strawberries or small bunch of grapes

A portion of vegetables can be:

■ A bowl of salad

■ tablespoons of cooked vegetables

supplemental help

A few supplements may help you reach your goals more quickly:

■ **Protein-carbohydrate shakes**: Getting all your nutrients from food can be difficult, especially when you're following an intense training programme and don't have enough time to prepare meals from scratch. Protein-carbohydrate shakes can be a convenient way of topping up your food intake.

■ **Multivitamins and minerals**: Multivitamin and mineral supplements can act as insurance if you aren't getting enough nutrients from food. Antioxidant supplements containing beta-carotene, vitamin C, vitamin E, selenium, lycopene, and bioflavanoids may also be beneficial for promoting recovery and boosting immunity.

■ **Creatine**: For experienced athletes only, creatine may help increase your strength and muscle mass but it doesn't work for everyone. Recent research suggests lower daily doses (3–7 g) for 30 days give similar results as larger doses but with less risk of side-effects.

do's and don'ts

Do: Eat two to four hours before weights workouts. Good choices include porridge, cereal with milk, a chicken or cheese sandwich, a jacket potato with beans or pasta with tuna. Failing that, an apple, a few dried apricots, a handful of sultanas or a pot of yoghurt eaten 30 minutes beforehand will give you an energy boost and keep the shakes at bay.

Do: Have a drink and snack as soon as possible after your workout. Drink plenty of water to replenish fluid losses immediately after working out. Eat a carbohydrate- and protein-rich snack ideally within 30 minutes and no later than 2 hours. Try a couple of portions of fresh fruit with a pot of yoghurt; a tuna sandwich; a protein-carb shake; or a protein (sports) bar.

> **TIP**
>
> Aim for six to eight glasses of water daily and more during hot weather. Replenish fluid losses during exercise by drinking before, during and after your workout – add another 0.5–1 litre for every hour you exercise.

Do: Plan ahead. Eating every three or four hours requires building your day around eating. Schedule meals and take nutritious snacks and shakes with you if you have to eat on the go.

Don't: Skip meals. Leaving gaps of more than four hours between meals not only saps your energy but can also result in muscle loss as your body turns to protein for fuel. If you're busy, have smoothies, shakes, sandwiches, nuts and fruit to meet your nutritional needs.

Don't: Eat quick-fix foods. Fast foods, processed snacks and soft drinks are chock-a-block with sugar, saturated fat and salt – all great energy-sappers. They don't fill you up or satisfy your appetite so it's all too easy to passively over-consume calories.

Don't: Drink too much alcohol. Alcohol can encourage fat storage. It's high in calories, puts undue stress on the liver and can hinder your recovery after intense workouts. Stick to safe intakes – fewer than 21 weekly units for men and 14 for women (1 unit is half a pint of ordinary beer or a small glass of wine).

sample meal plan for building muscle

breakfast
1 cup (85 g) porridge oats
2 cups (400 ml) skimmed milk
1 handful (40 g) of raisins

morning snack
2 cartons (2 x 150 g) yoghurt

lunch
Tuna sandwiches (70 g tuna, 4 slices bread)
Salad with 1 tablespoon olive/ walnut/flaxseed oil
1 portion of fresh fruit

afternoon snack
1 protein-carb shake
1 portion of fresh fruit

evening meal
Chicken (85 g), vegetable and cashew stir-fry
85 g (dry weight) wholegrain rice

evening snack
4 rice crackers with 4 tablespoons cottage cheese
2 portions of fresh fruit

daily totals
2750 Calories
125 g protein
436 g carbohydrate
56 g fat

6 maintenance

Congratulations on reaching the end of this six-week programme! Hopefully, you have now achieved your initial goals and are pleased with your results.

moving on

The programme has introduced you to new exercises, and helped you to establish new diet and activity habits. But the programme doesn't end just because the book does. Give yourself a short break from the plan – I suggest a week – then decide on your next goal. You can either repeat the programme or incorporate any of the exercises into a longer-term workout and diet plan to maintain your better body and your overall fitness.

Stick to the following principles:

- Aim to complete three weights and three CV workouts each week.

- You can choose whether to repeat the two-way split workout (weeks 3 and 4, see pages 29–45) or the three-way split workout (weeks 4 and 5, pages 46–72).

- Change your workout at least every four to six weeks to avoid training plateaux, to continue making muscle and strength gains, and to increase your motivation.

- Vary your CV activity as often as possible to increase your calorie burn, boost your motivation and reduce injury risk.

- Make sure you push yourself hard enough every workout.

- To avoid over-training, do not train a muscle group more than twice a week, and have at least one rest day per week.

- Re-read 'Training Tips' (pages 5–7) to ensure you always use good technique and don't lapse into bad habits.

- Continue to eat smart – re-read the tips in Chapter 5.

Best wishes and good luck!

index

alcohol 99

back extension 26
back extension with rotation 72
back problems 9
ball, exercise 8
barbell bench press 30
bench press machine 20
bent-over barbell row 50
bent-over lateral raise 58
body fat percentage 2
    body fat monitor 2
    skinfold callipers 2
body measurement log 3

cable crossover 49
cable lateral raise 57
calf stretch 14
calories 96
carbohydrates 97
cardiovascular (CV) exercise 74–5
chest/biceps stretch 16
circuit training 18
compound exercises 18
concentration curl 60
concentric exercise 6, 10
core training 7
    core stability 7
crunch 54

dead lift 67
dorsal raise 45
dumbbell curl 22
dumbbell flye 48
dumbbell shoulder press 34, 56

eccentric exercise 6, 10
exercise ball crunch 27
exercise ball pull-in 70
exercises, weeks five and six 46–72
exercises, weeks one and two 29–45
exercises, weeks three and four 46–62
EZ bar curl 59

fat 9
fat burning 73–5
fat burning workouts 78–80
    advanced interval 80
    beginners' steady pace 78
    intermediate interval 79

flexibility 9, 10
five-a-day 97–8
fruit 97–8

goal setting 2

hamstring stretch 14
hanging leg raise 64
heart rate monitor 76
heart rate training zones 75
    maximal heart rate (MHR) 75–6
    target heart rate training guide 75–6
hip and outer thigh stretch 14
hip flexor stretch 14

incline barbell bench press 47
incline dumbbell bench press 31
incline dumbbell curl 36
interval training 75

joints 10
    stability 18

lat pull-down 51
leg curls on the ball 40
leg extension 68
leg press 19
lifting belts 9
lower back stretch 14
lying triceps extension 37

machine row 21
machine squat 66
meal plan 100
motivation 2
    partner training 4
    rewards 4
    personal trainers 5
muscles 8
bulk 11
endurance 18

neck stretch 15
nutrition 95–100
    guidelines 95

one-legged dumbbell
        calf raise 28
overhead machine press 25

perceived exertion (PE) 76
    rating of (RPE) 77
Pilates 7
posture
good 7
    neutral 7
protein requirements 96–7
pull-up machine 32
pyramid training 6

reverse crunch 53
reverse-grip triceps
        press-down 61
reverse lunge 41
resistance training   vii
rest 10

seated cable row 33
seated inner thigh stretch 13
seated overhead triceps extension 62
sets training 29
    pyramid training method 29
    sets based workout 29
    three-way split 46
two-way split 29

shoulder stretch 16
side bridge 44
side crunch 71
split squat 39
standing calf raise 42
standing front thigh stretch 13
standing inner thigh stretch 13
straight arm pull-downs 52
straight leg dead lift 69
strength 18
step-ups 24
stretching 12–17
supplements 98

training tempo 6, 10
training terms 4
    one-rep max (1RM) 4
    overload 4
repetitions 4
rest interval 4
    sets 4
triceps dip 23
triceps stretch 17
twisting crunch 63
twisting exercise ball crunch 43

upper back stretch 16
upright row 35

vegetables 97–8
visualisation 4

warm up 5, 14
water 99
weight gain 96
workout logs 81–93
workout rules 17